T0185888

Near Misses in Cardiac Surgery

Thoralf M. Sundt · Duke E. Cameron ·
Myles E. Lee
Editors

Near Misses in Cardiac Surgery

Second Edition

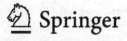

Editors
Thoralf M. Sundt
Massachusetts General Hospital
Boston, MA, USA

Duke E. Cameron
Massachusetts General Hospital
Boston, MA, USA

Myles E. Lee
Centinela Hospital Medical Center
Inglewood, CA, USA

ISBN 978-3-030-92752-3   ISBN 978-3-030-92750-9   (eBook)
https://doi.org/10.1007/978-3-030-92750-9

1st edition: © Myles Edwin Lee 2008
2nd edition: © The Editor(s) (if applicable) and The Author(s), under exclusive license to Springer Nature Switzerland AG 2022

This work is subject to copyright. All rights are solely and exclusively licensed by the Publisher, whether the whole or part of the material is concerned, specifically the rights of translation, reprinting, reuse of illustrations, recitation, broadcasting, reproduction on microfilms or in any other physical way, and transmission or information storage and retrieval, electronic adaptation, computer software, or by similar or dissimilar methodology now known or hereafter developed.

The use of general descriptive names, registered names, trademarks, service marks, etc. in this publication does not imply, even in the absence of a specific statement, that such names are exempt from the relevant protective laws and regulations and therefore free for general use.

The publisher, the authors and the editors are safe to assume that the advice and information in this book are believed to be true and accurate at the date of publication. Neither the publisher nor the authors or the editors give a warranty, expressed or implied, with respect to the material contained herein or for any errors or omissions that may have been made. The publisher remains neutral with regard to jurisdictional claims in published maps and institutional affiliations.

This Springer imprint is published by the registered company Springer Nature Switzerland AG
The registered company address is: Gewerbestrasse 11, 6330 Cham, Switzerland

With affection and respect to the memory of Philip N. Sawyer, MD, who initiated me into the rites, to the memory of David Preston Boyd, MD, who illuminated my path, and to Allison Elizabeth, Evan Preston, and Ladybug, who give relevance to everything that is good and worth a struggle.

Myles E. Lee

And to the patients who place their lives in our hands, the trainees who accept the challenge of the specialty, to our colleagues who support us as a team, and to the less visible members of the team, our families, who unselfishly make the sacrifices necessary to support us through the lows associated with our "near misses" and even harder through our "hits."

Thoralf M. Sundt and Duke E. Cameron

Foreword

A contemporary medical novelist, who is also a physician, once asked me if anything ever happened in the operating room that instantly changed the environment from quiet solitude to a life-threatening crisis. Experienced cardiac surgeons will surely smile at that question. The example that I provided to my novelist friend was acute aortic dissection during cannulation for cardiopulmonary bypass. Such an event demonstrates that the exhortation, "The best way to treat complications is to avoid them," is not always possible.

Since the advent of open-heart surgery some 70 years ago, the need to respond immediately and effectively to such life-threatening events has resulted in the perplexing tendency to describe surgeons, especially cardiac surgeons, as being courageous. However, a popular modern philosopher, G. K. Chesterton (1874–1936), defined courage as "…. a strong desire to live taking the form of a readiness to die." While cardiac surgeons routinely face the responsibility of treating patients who clearly desire to live but risk the real possibility of dying, the surgeon is at no imminent risk of death. Thus, it seems more appropriate to speak of "courageous patients" than of "courageous surgeons." Nevertheless, more than any other practitioners of medicine, cardiac surgeons can too often converse normally with a patient in the morning and pronounce that patient dead on the same afternoon. Since the only intervening event in such instances is the surgical procedure, cardiac surgeons have a moral responsibility to exert maximum effort at developing their skills. Obviously, those skills include manual dexterity but perhaps more importantly, they also include the ability to avoid problems and to deal with them quickly and efficiently when they occur. Mistakes, "near misses," are often more instructive than event-free successes, but the latter are usually forgotten. However, "near misses" are never forgotten.

These simple, rather banal, truths explain why the first edition of "Near Misses in Cardiac Surgery" by Dr. Myles Lee, first published nearly 30 years ago, quickly became a must-read for a generation of cardiac surgeons. Myles Lee is a superb cardiac surgeon with all the gifts of manual dexterity, knowledge of his subject, and the ability to convey that knowledge to his peers. The art of teaching is simply the ability to transfer the information in the teacher's mind to the mind of the student.

There are multiple techniques for accomplishing that task and the approach utilized by Dr. Lee in "Near Misses in Cardiac Surgery" has proven to be highly effective. An actual clinical case of a surviving patient is presented, and the patient's problem is posed to the reader, who is faced with determining the cause of the problem and solving it before the patient's demise. After giving the reader this opportunity, the clinical problem is then identified, and its actual resolution is revealed. Each case presentation concludes with a detailed discussion and references. Thus, the reader is challenged to act as if the fate of each patient depends on his or her ability to make appropriate decisions quickly and under pressure before tragedy strikes, a familiar real-world situation for all cardiac surgeons.

"Near Misses in Cardiac Surgery" was first published in 1992, and an edition was reissued in 2009. It is now being updated under the guidance of new co-editors, Dr. Thoralf M. Sundt III and Dr. Duke E. Cameron, two of the most respected and admired cardiac surgeons in our profession. Dr. Sundt is Churchill Professor of Surgery at Harvard and Chief of the Division of Cardiac Surgery at the Massachusetts General Hospital in Boston. Dr. Cameron, Former Professor and Chief of Cardiac Surgery at Johns Hopkins University in Baltimore, is currently a colleague of Dr. Sundt's as Professor of Surgery at Harvard, Co-Director of the Thoracic Aortic Center at Massachusetts General Hospital. Both new editors are Past-Presidents of the American Association for Thoracic Surgery, a testament to the esteem in which they are held by their peers. This second edition of "Near Misses in Cardiac Surgery" is more than worthy of the high standard set by the first edition. It includes multiple new clinical cases and of course updated modern solutions and references to the problems posed. This new edition is once again a must-read for all professionals who are involved or interested in modern cardiac surgery.

Chicago, Illinois, USA   James L. Cox, MD
October 2021

Preface

With its emphasis on teamwork, interdisciplinary communication, anticipation of next steps, standardization and simplicity of techniques, and unflagging vigilance for the unexpected, *Near Misses in Cardiac Surgery*, in print since 1992, created a real-time atmosphere in which a nonjudgmental approach to problem-solving in adverse circumstances, often with incomplete information, facilitated the conversion of experience into corrective action. Written in the second-person present tense, and knowing in advance that all the patients survived, the reader, as surgeon, experienced the terror and anguish of confronting unexpected difficulties that if not immediately corrected would have resulted in the patient's demise.

Advances in surgical techniques, such as off-pump procedures, mini-invasive incisions, and robotic surgery, as well as catheter-based methods to replace valves, close inter-chamber septal defects, and repair aortic aneurysms performed by interventionalists in hybrid operating rooms, have only heightened the need to recognize teamwork and communication, anticipation, standardization, and vigilance.

My goal, to paraphrase Kipling, was to enable readers to keep their heads "when all about you are losing theirs and blaming it on you." I learned on my first day in medical school that "you are responsible for the skin and its contents." That is when I decided to become an internist who operates. This approach lent credence to my belief that decisions, based upon the ability to apply accumulated knowledge, are more important than incisions. The surgical and non-surgical lessons internalized from each patient interaction provide the confidence that enables us to make the best decisions and function in stressful situations while transferring equanimity to others in the operating room. I must confess it was more enjoyable to write about these experiences than to live through them (it is not only the patient who goes home with scars!). Clearly, surgeons do not play God. God does not sweat the way we do.

Our patients exhibit great courage and trust as they face the unknown, often at the mercy of strangers. As Theodore Roosevelt said, "no one cares how much you know until they know how much you care." Our obligation is to assure them of the safest passage through uncharted waters. In this sense, we must never follow our patients. We must lead them.

Inglewood, USA   Myles E. Lee

During recent years, as Duke Cameron and I have had the good fortune to work in the same unit, we have had found more and more things in common, one of which is our high regard for Dr. Lee's original text. We have found it a remarkably useful tool educating ourselves and our residents, filling a niche not quite satisfied by the standard texts in our specialty. The book was engaging both for the literary style in which Dr. Lee described the cases and the practical relevance of each scenario. It was, in fact, following a near miss in our practice that we looked at one another and remarked how useful it would be to our trainees if *near misses* were updated to reflect contemporary practice. We were delighted when Dr. Lee was receptive and so began a delightful journey to create a second edition making every effort to preserve the attributes of brevity, relevance, and honesty that characterize the original work.

It is our earnest hope that readers will find this version as engaging and useful as we found the original. Cardiac surgery is a complex endeavor in which accidents are, at some level, inevitable as it is the case for other such industries. A great deal has been written about error prevention with tools such as checklists, but a more comprehensive approach to error management as has been adopted by other high-risk, high-consequence industries must include error capture and recovery. This book focuses on error capture through vigilance and error recovery through teamwork, a territory less crowed in our literature. We have all made mistakes in our clinical practices. Meaning can be derived from those errors—and their consequences—if we learn from them ourselves and share those learnings with others.

Boston, USA   Thoralf M. Sundt
                                                                     Duke E. Cameron

Acknowledgements

When Dr. Sundt and Dr. Cameron approached me with their proposal to not only update *Near Misses in Cardiac Surgery* but to add numerous cases from their own voluminous archives, I was relieved to learn I had not been alone all these years. I feel honored to share the arena with surgeons of their stature who saw fit to pick up where I left off. I wish to acknowledge all my past colleagues, men and women of erudition, skill, courage, tenacity, and indefatigability, upon whose shoulders I have stood and from whom I learned everything.

Dr. Lee

Contents

Acronyms

ACT	Activated clotting time
ARDS	Acute respiratory distress syndrome
AS	Aortic stenosis
ASA score	American Society of Anesthesiologists Physical Status Score
AV	Atrio-ventricular groove dissociation
AVM	Arteriovenous malformation
AVR	Aortic valve replacement
BMI	Body mass index
BSA	Body surface area
CABG x3	Three-vessel coronary artery bypass graft operation
CCU	Cardiac care unit
CO	Cardiac output
COPD	Chronic obstructive pulmonary disease
CT	Computed tomography
CTA	Computed tomographic angiogram
CTEPH	Chronic thromboembolic pulmonary hypertension
CVP	Central venous pressure
CXR	Chest X-ray
DVT	Deep venous thrombosis
eCPR	Extracorporeal cardiopulmonary resuscitation
ED/ER	Emergency department/emergency room
EKG	Echocardiogram
EOPA(r)	Elongated One-Piece Arterial Cannula
Esmark	Esmark dressing; Esmark with Ioban dressing
HCT	Hematocrit
Heyde syndrome	Multisystem disorder: aortic stenosis, gastrointestinal bleeding; acquired von Willebrand syndrome
HIT/HITT	Heparin-induced thrombocytopenia (HIT) and thrombosis (HITT)
HOCM	Hypertrophic obstructive cardiomyopathy
IABP	Intra-aortic balloon pump

ICD	Implantable cardioverter-defibrillator
ICU	Intensive care unit
IMA	Internal mammary artery
INR	International normalized ratio (PTT/INR)
ITA	Internal thoracic artery
IVC	Inferior vena cava
IVUS	Intravascular ultrasound
LAD	Left anterior descending
LAO	Left anterior oblique
LIMA	Left internal mammary artery
LITA	Left internal thoracic artery
LVAD	Left ventricular assist device
MAC	Mitral annular calcification
MAP	Mean arterial pressure
MVO2	Myocardial oxygen consumption
MVR	Mitral valve replacement
NT-proBNP	N-terminal (NT-pro hormone BNP
OHT	Orthotopic heart transplant
OM	Obtuse marginal artery
OM1	Ostial lesion
OM2	Ostial lesion
P1, P2	Scallop
PA	Physician assistant
PA	Pulmonary artery
PAPi	Pulmonary arterial pulsatility index
PCI	Percutaneous coronary intervention
PCWP	Pulmonary capillary wedge pressure
PDA	Posterior descending artery
PEA	Pulseless electrical activity
PEEP	Positive end expiratory pressure
PFO	Patent foramen ovale
PPM	Permanent pacemaker
PTT	Prothrombin time
PVR	Pulmonary vascular resistance
PVR	Pulse volume recording, i.e., blood pressure cuffs
RAO	Right anterior oblique, e.g., cranial projection
RCA	Right coronary artery
RFV	Right femoral vein
RIJ	Right internal jugular
ROSC	Return of spontaneous circulation
RV	Right ventricle
SA	Sinoatrial node
SAM	Systolic anterior motion
SBP	Systolic blood pressure
SH needle	Stands for small half circle needle

SMA	Superior mesenteric artery
STEMI	ST elevated myocardial infarction
SVC	Superior vena cava
SVG	Saphenous vein graft
TACO	Transfusion-associated circulatory overload
TEE	Transesophageal echocardiogram
TEVAR	Thoracic endovascular aortic repair
TRALI	Transfusion-associated lung injury
VA-ECMO	Veno-arterial extracoproeal membrane oxygenation
VV-ECMO	Veno-venous extracoproeal membrane oxygenation

Chapter 1
Aortic Cannulation

Jordan P. Bloom, Myles E. Lee, and Arminder S. Jassar

Problem

The sun's golden crest is just visible over the mountain tops as you bound out of bed and head for the hospital on an empty freeway enchanted by a Chopin nocturne. You will operate on a 45-year-old man with an 8-year history of exertional angina. He had exercise-induced anterior segment wall motion abnormalities, a positive exercise thallium study, and angiographic confirmation of a long muscle bridge overlying the midportion of the left anterior descending coronary artery. Except for some ventricular apical akinesis, cardiac function is normal. Medical therapy, which included beta-blockers and calcium channel blockers, had failed to relieve the symptoms. Dividing a muscle bridge? A resident's case!

At surgery, the aorta was slightly smaller than expected for a 75 kg patient. Nonetheless, you palpate the aorta to identify a soft spot and perform your standard aortic cannulation using a 20 Fr EOPA arterial cannula at the level of the pericardial reflection. You observe normal pulsatile back bleeding through the aortic cannula upon de-airing, and the line pressure correlates with the radial arterial pressure. The right atrium was cannulated using a 29/37 Fr dual stage venous cannula and an aortic root vent/cardioplegia cannula was placed uneventfully. After performing the pre-bypass checklist, cardiopulmonary bypass is commenced. The drainage appears adequate, and you ask the perfusionist to drift to 34 °C for an anticipated short case.

J. P. Bloom · A. S. Jassar (✉)
Department of Surgery, Massachusetts General Hospital, Boston, MA, USA
e-mail: ajassar@mgh.harvard.edu

J. P. Bloom
e-mail: jpbloom@mgh.harvard.edu

M. E. Lee
Cardiothoracic Surgery, Centinela Hospital Medical Center, Inglewood, CA, USA

© The Author(s), under exclusive license to Springer Nature Switzerland AG 2022
T. M. Sundt et al. (eds.), *Near Misses in Cardiac Surgery*,
https://doi.org/10.1007/978-3-030-92750-9_1

1

As you elevate the heart from the pericardium to identify the LAD, the perfusionist casually informs you that she cannot maintain a flow rate of more than 1.8 L/min/m^2 due to high arterial inflow pressure despite a right radial arterial line pressure of only 34 mmHg. You let the heart down back into the pericardial space. You do your best to inspect the aorta. True, there was a subadventitial hematoma at the cannulation site as sometimes happens, but now it seems more extensive. You tell yourself you have seen this before without complications, but in your heart, you know what this is; you just cannot believe it is happening to this healthy young patient, who was the very first from a new referral source, and on such a bright sunny morning.

Solution

You immediately ask the anesthesiologist to interrogate the aorta for potential dissection using transesophageal echocardiography. They confirm your worst fears and report a dissection flap in the descending aorta. The dissection flap involves the ascending aorta and extends into the sinus segment, causing mild-to-moderate aortic regurgitation. Since you are unable to adequately flow on cardiopulmonary bypass, your first priority is to establish alternative arterial cannulation. You have not yet arrested the heart, so you wean from bypass and expeditiously perform a groin incision to expose the femoral artery, which thankfully does not appear dissected. You carefully cannulate the femoral artery, switch perfusion to the new cannula, and gradually resume cardiopulmonary bypass. The perfusionist informs you that they can flow a rate of 2.4 L/min/m^2 with normal line pressures. Now that you have adequate bypass flow, you begin to cool the patient to 18 °C in preparation for circulatory arrest. When the heart fibrillates, you cross clamp the aorta and deliver retrograde cardioplegia. You open the ascending aorta through a transverse incision and notice the dissection flap that extends distally into the area of the cross-clamp. You identify the coronary ostia and carefully provide additional cardioplegia directly into the coronary arteries using ostial cardioplegia catheters and achieve a quick diastolic arrest. You carefully examine the aortic root. The dissection flap extends into the non-coronary sinus but does not involve the left or right coronary sinuses, or the coronary ostia. You are relieved to see there are no intimal tears in the root. You prepare the proximal aorta for anastomosis at the level of the sinotubular junction using a "felt sandwich" technique, attaching strips of Teflon felt both inside and outside the aorta using a loosely run prolene suture. While you continue to cool, you perform the unroofing of the LAD myocardial bridge, which by now has become an "incidental" portion of the operation. Once the patient is at 18 °C, you halt the cardiopulmonary bypass, remove the cross-clamp, and examine the aortic lumen. This enables you to identify a 1 cm laceration in the posterior wall of the ascending aorta at the level of the aortic cannula. You are relieved to see that the intimal tear is limited to the ascending aorta and does not extend into the aortic arch. You resect the entirety of the intimal tear and perform a beveled hemiarch anastomosis proximal to the innominate artery. After the distal anastomosis is constructed, bypass is resumed via the side branch of the graft. The line pressures are low, and radial pressure matches the central aortic pressure. Rewarming is initiated and you take a deep breath. The remainder of the operation is completed uneventfully.

Discussion

The incidence of intraoperative aortic dissection originating in the ascending aorta is 0.06–0.16%, [1, 2] but carries a mortality rate of up to 48% [2]. The most common etiology in the past was intimal injury caused by a partial occlusion clamp, but dissections have been known to occur anywhere the aorta is manipulated, including cannulation sites or proximal anastomosis sites for vein grafts. The risk of perioperative dissections is reduced by avoiding multiple clamp applications and lowering aortic pressure around the time of cannulation and clamp application and removal. The aortic dissection in this case was caused by the tip of the aortic cannula that injured the posterior wall of the aorta. The initial back bleeding was reassuring; however, with the initiation of cardiopulmonary bypass, what was initially just a localized tear became a full dissection. The first sign of an iatrogenic aortic dissection may be an unexpected rise in the aortic perfusion pressure and diminished bypass flow rates. Based on patterns of regional malperfusion, this can be accompanied by a drop in measured arterial line pressure, despite a tense aorta in the field. Dissection may be apparent on gross inspection of the ascending aorta and the aortic arch, although distinguishing this from the more common limited sub-adventitial hematoma can sometimes be challenging. The definitive diagnosis in the current era is most commonly made by transesophageal echocardiography. While the views of the aortic arch may be limited by the left main stem bronchus, TEE provides excellent visualization of the ascending and descending aorta and can confirm the diagnosis.

In this case, the dissection becomes apparent upon commencing bypass but before stopping the heart, permitting you to wean from bypass to allow antegrade perfusion from the heart, while an alternate arterial cannulation site is prepared. If the dissection had become apparent only after the heart was already arrested, an alternate cannulation would need to be quickly established and the arterial perfusion line switched to support the circulation. The options for arterial cannulation in this situation include another site of the ascending aorta or one of its branches (e.g., innominate artery), the right axillary artery, or the femoral artery. Even in the presence of an acute dissection, the ascending aorta can be cannulated over a wire placed into the true lumen as confirmed by TEE. This technique requires familiarity, both on the surgeon's and the echocardiographer's part. While right axillary artery cannulation has the advantage of facilitating selective cerebral perfusion during circulatory arrest, it may not always be prepped into the field and generally takes longer to establish than femoral cannulation. Most surgeons favor the femoral artery which can be cannulated expeditiously via either percutaneous or open approaches. Some have advocated cannulation via the left ventricular apex, although this is not commonly performed. LV apex cannulation is not an option if the aorta has already been cross clamped. Also, even if performed prior to aortic clamping, it precludes clamping the aorta in the presence of significant aortic regurgitation. Arterial inflow can be switched by briefly discontinuing cardiopulmonary bypass, placing clamps on the aortic inflow cannula, dividing the line, and reconnecting into the new inflow cannula; this could be completed in less than 30 s with careful attention to adequate de-airing before reinitiating bypass. Panic is the enemy here. A similar approach can be applied if dissection occurs with removal of the cross-clamp, for example, after a coronary bypass operation. In this situation one can expect the ascending aorta to turn blue, but most dramatically, each proximal venous bypass anastomosis will start bleeding profusely as the sutures loosen with proximal progression of the dissection.

While local repairs were advocated in the past, in the current era, graft replacement of the involved proximal aorta with complete excision of the area of intimal injury is recommended. In this case, because you are not sure of the origin of the dissection, which could be at the cannulation site or at the site of the antegrade cardioplegia catheter, circulatory arrest allows a thorough examination of the aortic lumen to identify the site of injury. Adjunct retrograde or selective antegrade cerebral perfusion can be used based on the surgeon's experience. Similarly, techniques for conducting circulatory arrest at moderate hypothermia have been described and can be employed based on surgeon experience and preference. The distal anastomosis can be performed as a hemi-arch replacement or as a zone 1 arch replacement between the carotid and innominate arteries depending on the location of the tear. In all instances bypass should be reinitiated antegrade via a side arm of the ascending aortic graft. If reimplantation of the innominate artery is required, a 12- or 14-mm graft can be sewn end-to-end to the stump of the innominate and end-to-side to the ascending graft at least 2–3 cm proximal to the distal anastomosis, affording a stable landing zone for endovascular repair should subsequent distal interventions be required.

References

1. Still RJ, Hilgenberg AD, Akins CW, Daggett WM, Buckley MJ. Intraoperative aortic dissection. Ann Thorac Surg. 1992;53(3):374–80.
2. Williams ML, Sheng S, Gammie JS, Rankin JS, Smith PK, Hughes GC. Aortic dissection as a complication of cardiac surgery: report from the society of thoracic surgeons database. Ann Thorac Surg. 2010;90(6):1812–7.

Chapter 2
Return to the Operating Room

Myles E. Lee

Problem

A 75-year-old patient has been evaluated by his cardiologist because of the recent onset of exertional chest discomfort. Although the symptoms are mild, the patient undergoes a treadmill test, which not only reproduces his symptoms at low level of activity but is also associated with hypotension, 4 mm precordial ST segment depression with a prolonged recovery phase, and frequent premature ventricular contractions. At cardiac catheterization there is good left ventricular contractility with an ejection fraction of 55%. There is subtotal obstruction of the left main coronary artery and total obstruction of the right coronary artery that fills distally through left-to-right transseptal collaterals. The patient has had no major prior illnesses, takes no medications, and has no allergies. Your preoperative evaluation includes a duplex scan of the carotid arteries, revealing mild plaquing with no flow disturbances in the internal carotid arteries, and a scan of the saphenous veins reveals them to be patent and of a diameter suitable for use as conduits.

At surgery, you perform routine cannulations, including a right atrial cannula for the administration of retrograde cardioplegia. You begin cardiopulmonary bypass by placing vein grafts to the circumflex and right coronary arteries, then graft the left internal thoracic artery to the midportion of the left anterior descending coronary artery. Separation from bypass is uneventful and the grafts lay perfectly. You place right atrial and right ventricular pacing wires and leave tubes in the left pleural space, the anterior mediastinum, and the posterior pericardium.

Once in the intensive care unit the patient has normal hemodynamics and good blood gases, with virtually no drainage from the chest tubes. You feel virtually

M. E. Lee (✉)
Department of Cardiothoracic Surgery, Centinela Hospital Medical Center, Inglewood, CA, USA

© The Author(s), under exclusive license to Springer Nature Switzerland AG 2022
T. M. Sundt et al. (eds.), *Near Misses in Cardiac Surgery*,
https://doi.org/10.1007/978-3-030-92750-9_2

5

blessed that this patient has done so well because 6 months ago you captured two press row tickets in the center orchestra section for tonight's percformance of "Phantom of the Opera," a phenomenon that has always been sold out a year in advance, and you will not be denied what after today you believe will be a just award.

The auctioneer has just illuminated the restored chandelier from the old Paris Opera house. There is an enormous flash as the fortissimo tones of the overture reverberate through your body. Riveted to your seat, you gaze in astonishment as the chandelier rises, swinging and glittering from the stage, suspended, swaying for a moment a few feet above the floor before lurching out over the audience. Surely this chandelier is going to land in your lap! But at the last possible moment, it veers sharply upward to complete its ascent to the rafters of the theater. Almost immediately, the massive set from Chalumeau's "Hannibal" unfolds, flanking the stage with two massive stone idols 40 feet high. Carlotta has begun her Aria when you feel the first tiny vibration at the level of your left hip. But it is not Carlotta's Aria you feel. It is a beeper call from the intensive care unit.

Benumbed, you slink out of the theater to the harsh luminescence of the telephone booth where you learn that your patient's blood pressure has suddenly crashed. The nurses tell you that the filling pressures have been low for much of the evening and that the patient has required more than the usual amount of volume replacement. There has been only insignificant drainage from the chest tubes and the abdomen is not distended. They tell you that a repeat chest roentgenogram looks quite different from the normal postoperative film you saw a few hours earlier, and that you had better come in right away. You slide back to your seat, clamber over half the row of annoyed patrons, press some taxi money into the hand of your loving spouse, trample the patrons a third time, and head to the hospital.

Solution

The magic glow of the evening is quickly replaced by the fluorescent glare of the chest film thrust onto the view box. There is a white-out of the right pleural space. You can hear some air entering into the right lung and there is no mediastinal shift suggestive of volume loss. You cannot believe it, but there is a very large right pleural effusion. Confirmatory evidence is provided by the filling pressures which are in the 2–3 mmHg range, and by the patient's hematocrit which is 15%. At surgery, the pericardium is dry. There is not a clot to be seen. All the grafts are patent. You do notice a little pool of blood that keeps welling up from underneath the lower aspect of the right half of the sternum. On closer inspection you see a tiny pumper in the mediastinal fat ejecting blood with mocking precision directly into a 2 mm hole in the right mediastinal pleura. After ligating the bleeder, you open the pleural space widely and then evacuate a lake of warm blood (enough that the Phantom could have filled the lagoon in the bowels of the Paris Opera House perhaps 10 times over) into the Cell Saver. You inspect the pleural space for other surprises, such as the tip of an intravenous catheter, and examine the visceral pleura for evidence of subpleural hemorrhage caused by an over-wedged Swan-Ganz pulmonary artery catheter. Finding neither, you place an additional chest tube in the right pleural space and close the incision.

Discussion

This case illustrates one of those perverse, infuriating, unpredictable, unreportable, anecdotal events that can easily mar an otherwise uncomplicated procedure, not to mention a once-in-a-lifetime evening. Of course, the offending vessel was not bleeding at the closure of the initial procedure and had to have been in spasm. The hole in the right mediastinal pleura had to have been made during the creation of the T-incision in the inferior pericardium and it was hidden by the mediastinal fat. It was remarkable that the bleeding vessel could evacuate itself directly into this hole and nowhere else. It was equally remarkable in the sense of being commendable that the intensive care unit nurses had the insight to order a chest film to help define a puzzling clinical situation. They had expected to find volume accumulation in the left pleural space, related to the dissection of the left internal thoracic artery, with the assumption that the left pleura was clotted preventing its evacuation. This is a prime example of the teamwork necessary for superior results. This case also illustrates the necessity for prompt action based on information at hand, incomplete and incomprehensible though it be, rather than hesitation based on denials that just because you cannot come up with the immediate explanation, it just cannot be.

Postoperative hemorrhage is associated with significant morbidity both in the short-term and long-term. Interventions such as hemostasis checklists have been introduced in an effort to minimize this complication. In this case despite best efforts, hemorrhage ensued. Cardiac surgery is a complex endeavor with multiple potential pitfalls.

Bibliography

1. Dyke C, Aronson S, Dietrich W, Hofmann A, Karkouti K, Levi M, Murphy GJ, Sellke FW, Shore-Lesserson L, von Heymann C, Ranucci M. Universal definition of perioperative bleeding in adult cardiac surgery. J Thorac Cardiovasc Surg. 2014;147(5):1458–63.e1. 0.1016/j. jtcvs.2013.10.070. Epub 2013 Dec 9. PMID: 24332097 F.
2. Ali JM, Gerrard C, Clayton J, Moorjani N. Hemostasis checklist reduces bleeding and blood product consumption after cardiac surgery. Ann Thorac Surg. 2021;111(5):1570–7. https://doi. org/10.1016/j.athoracsur.2020.07.016 Epub 2020 Sep 19. PMID: 32956672.
3. Karthik S, Grayson AD, McCarron EE, Pullan DM, Desmond MJ. Reexploration for bleeding after coronary artery bypass surgery: risk factors, outcomes, and the effect of time delay. Ann Thorac Surg. 2004;78(2):527–34; discussion 534. https://doi.org/10.1016/j.athoracsur.2004.02. 088. PMID: 15276512.

4. Jakobsen CJ, Ryhammer PK, Tang M, Andreasen JJ, Mortensen PE. Transfusion of blood during cardiac surgery is associated with higher long-term mortality in low-risk patients. Eur J Cardiothorac Surg. 2012;42(1):114–20. https://doi.org/10.1093/ejcts/ezr242 Epub 2012 Jan 12. PMID: 22241009.

Chapter 3
Cannulation for ECMO

John M. Trahanas and Jerome C. Crowley

Problem

Having just finished Saturday morning rounds, you are about to exit the hospital to a beautiful spring day addressing your "honey-do" list when your pager goes off. It's the cardiology ICU, asking you to come evaluate an obese 19-year-old man with viral myocarditis and escalating pharmacologic support requirements. You could ask them to page the on-call surgeon to come in from home, but as you are right downstairs you head up to assess the situation.

When you arrive in the ICU, you find a patient with cold extremities and escalating norepinephrine requirements. The intensivist shows you a trans-thoracic echo (TTE) from several hours prior which reveals severe biventricular dysfunction. The patient has rapidly progressed to substantial doses of inotropes and pressor agents with marginal hemodynamic improvement, and his rising lactic acid and worsening liver and kidney function speak to the failure of medical management. While you stand there, you witness several salvos of non-sustained ventricular tachycardia with almost no pulse pressure on the arterial line. So much for bringing your colleague in from home. The time to act is now.

You call for the ECMO team. Soon the ICU is flooded with OR nurses and equipment. You prep and drape the patient's groins and chest, choose your cannulas, and bring the ECMO lines up. Under ultrasound guidance you obtain percutaneous access to the right femoral vein, antegrade access to the right superficial femoral artery, and retrograde access to the right common femoral artery. You give heparin and place a distal perfusor in the superficial femoral artery without issue. You choose a Super Stiff wire for the vein, and it seems to advance smoothly to

J. M. Trahanas
Department of Surgery, Vanderbilt University, Nashville, TN, USA

J. C. Crowley (✉)
Department of Anesthesia, Massachusetts General Hospital, Boston, MA, USA
e-mail: jccrowley@mgh.harvard.edu

© The Author(s), under exclusive license to Springer Nature Switzerland AG 2022
T. M. Sundt et al. (eds.), *Near Misses in Cardiac Surgery*,
https://doi.org/10.1007/978-3-030-92750-9_3

40 cm. The trans-esophageal echo (TEE) probe has not yet arrived, so you place your TTE probe on the chest and attempt to visualize the inferior vena cava. You see what you think is the vessel (it is dilated consistent with cardiogenic shock), but you can't see your wire. A soft J wire passes easily from the femoral artery and is readily seen in the descending aorta. You are not an expert echocardiographer, and the vibrations of your mobile phone (undoubtedly your spouse wondering where you are) tempt you to cannulate the vessel regardless of not being able to find the wire. You resist, knowing the right thing to do is to wait for definitive imaging while the patient still has a pulse.

Solution

The TEE probe arrives, and the cardiac intensivist confirms there is no wire in the inferior vena cava or the right atrium. When they push the probe in distally, the wire cannot be visualized as far as they can see. Perplexed, you withdraw your wire completely and make a new attempt to advance it into the vessel. Once again, you feel some resistance around 40 cm, which causes you to stop. You remove the Super Stiff wire and instead advance a flexible J wire which flutters easily into view in the right atrium on ultrasound. Relieved, you place a pigtail over the flexible J wire, and then exchange it for the Super Stiff wire. After serially dilating the venous tract, you then easily advance the venous ECMO cannula into the right atrium. You ask the intensivist to turn the view to the descending aorta, and after re-visualizing the flexible J wire in the aorta, you dilate and advance an appropriately sized arterial cannula. You go on veno-arterial ECMO and see an immediate improvement in hemodynamics. After breaking scrub and confirming the cannula position on plain film x-ray, you reach for your phone to answer the missed messages and are satisfied to see the drips start to melt away.

Discussion

Cannulation for veno-arterial or veno-venous ECMO is associated with technical and logistical challenges and is not without risk. Recognizing patients who are on a trajectory of clinical deterioration is important to ensure that cannulation occurs in a controlled environment, rather than in the chaos of a code event.

In a patient who is not in cardiac arrest, it is often easiest to place the distal perfusor before the re-infusion cannula, as the latter cannula blocks flow to the superficial femoral artery, making it more difficult to confirm arterial access. The presence of the larger arterial and venous cannulae also makes it more difficult to use ultrasound to obtain access for a distal perfusor.

Blind placement of ECMO cannulae should be avoided at all costs. Whenever possible, the venous wire should be visualized in the inferior vena cava/right atrium, and the arterial wire in the descending aorta. This helps to avoid the disastrous complication of vessel perforation that can occur when a cannula follows a misplaced wire to an unintended destination. Perforations can occur in the iliac vessels, the abdomen, the retro-hepatic vena cava, or in the chest, potentially leading to hemorrhagic shock, and depending on location, may require endovascular stenting or more commonly open exploration and repair.

The gold standard for cannulation is fluoroscopy; however, this is frequently not an option when cannulation occurs at the bedside. Trans-esophageal echocardiography can be obtained rapidly, and the bicaval view can confirm proper positioning of the venous wire. If a trans-esophageal probe or operator is not available, trans-thoracic echocardiography can also be used, with the subcostal view being the most effective for confirming wire placement.

For venous cannulation, especially in obese patients, a Super Stiff wire is preferred to avoid wire kinking in the subcutaneous tissues which also risks vessel perforation. When advancing a Super Stiff wire, it is important to stop at any sign of unexpected resistance, as the rigidity of the wire can easily perforate a vascular structure. When a Super Stiff wire does not pass easily, a flexible wire may suffice. Correct wire positioning in the right atrium can be obtained with the flexible wire and subsequently a pigtail catheter used to exchange to a Super Stiff wire for advancing the cannula.

One danger of using a soft wire for venous cannulation is that a kink in the wire near the tip of the wire may be missed and advanced into the patient; this could potentially deflect the cannula and cause a venous perforation, a devastating event in a patient requiring ECMO who would need emergent vascular surgery consultation, as well.

Bibliography

1. Julliard W, Teman N. Extracorporeal membrane oxygenation: how i teach it. Ann Thorac Surg. 2020;109:325–8.
2. Bisdas T, Beutel G, Warnecke G, Hoeper MM, Kuehn C, Haverich A, et al. Vascular complications in patients undergoing femoral cannulation for extracorporeal membrane oxygenation support. Ann Thorac Surg. 2011;92:626–31. https://doi.org/10.1016/j.athoracsur.2011.02.018.
3. Ramaiah C, Babu A. ECMO cannulation techniques. In: Extracorporeal membrane oxygenation-advances in therapy. IntechOpen;2016.
4. Banfi C, Pozzi M, Brunner M-E, Rigamonti F, Murith N, Mugnai D, et al. Veno-arterial extracorporeal membrane oxygenation: an overview of different cannulation techniques. J Thorac Dis. 2016;8:E875–85. https://doi.org/10.21037/jtd.2016.09.25.
5. Taslakian B, Ingber R, Aaltonen E, Horn J, Hickey R. Interventional radiology suite: a primer for trainees. J Clin Med. 2019;8:1347. https://doi.org/10.3390/jcm8091347.
6. Rupprecht L, Lunz D, Philipp A, Lubnow M, Schmid C. Pitfalls in percutaneous ECMO cannulation. Hear Lung Vessel. 2015;7:320.

Chapter 4
Transcatheter Aortic Valve Replacement (TAVR)

Asishana Osho and Nathaniel B. Langer

Problem

It is the end of a tough week, and you are quite pleased about the successful deployment of a transcatheter aortic valve (TAVR) in an 87-year-old woman with tortuous and calcified ilio-femoral vasculature. She had a left bundle branch block preoperatively but made it through the deployment without developing complete heart block. The delivery system was withdrawn without issue and the vessel was sealed using two percutaneous closure devices as is standard at your institution. Unfortunately, routine real time pulse volume recordings (PVR) obtained immediately after closing the access site now demonstrate a flat waveform on the deployment side. Preoperatively, the patient had normal waveforms bilaterally. You carefully elevate the drapes to verify that the PVR cuffs are appropriately placed. To your dismay the extremity of interest has taken on a dusky appearance, clearly indicating loss of peripheral perfusion.

Solution

You still have a wire in the contralateral femoral artery over which you pass a diagnostic catheter. The angiogram on the device side confirms your suspicion of a significant dissection of the common femoral artery at the access site. Using an omni-flush catheter you cross over to the dissected vessel and traverse the area of injury with a wire. Next you perform a balloon angioplasty at the site of dissection.

A. Osho · N. B. Langer (✉)
Department of Surgery, Massachusetts General Hospital, Boston, MA, USA
e-mail: Nlanger@partners.org

A. Osho
e-mail: Asishana.osho@mgh.harvard.edu

© The Author(s), under exclusive license to Springer Nature Switzerland AG 2022   13
T. M. Sundt et al. (eds.), *Near Misses in Cardiac Surgery*,
https://doi.org/10.1007/978-3-030-92750-9_4

Given evidence of a persistent dissection flap, you then place a covered stent over the area of injury. Your completion angiogram demonstrates excellent flow through the area of common femoral artery injury and good runoff to the distal vasculature. Follow-up PVRs demonstrate strong pulsatile waveforms bilaterally. The patient does well postoperatively and is discharged home two days after the procedure without claudication or other evidence of peripheral neurovascular insufficiency.

Discussion

The transfemoral approach to TAVR has been associated with superior outcomes and is most commonly used. However, given the sizeable diameter of sheaths required for valve positioning and deployment, injury to the ilio-femoral vasculature occurs in 10–20% of cases. Injury occurs most commonly at the access site in the common femoral artery but can occur at any location along the ilio-femoral vascular tree. Several studies have outlined a significant association between ilio-femoral complications and outcomes including mortality, length of stay, and post-TAVR quality of life. Fortunately, rates of ilio-femoral artery injury are decreasing as newer generations of devices are produced with improvements in sheath technology including steadily decreasing sheath sizes and modification of sheath properties to facilitate smooth intravascular passage.

Injury to ilio-femoral arteries during TAVR range in type and severity from access site hematomas and pseudoaneurysms, to arterial dissection and rupture. The latter two occur less frequently with estimated rates of 6.5% and 3.5%, respectively. Risk factors for ilio-femoral injury include patient factors (female gender, significant pelvic vessel calcifications, peripheral vascular disease), device factors (larger delivery systems, increased sheath-to-femoral artery ratio >1.05, failure of device closure), and operator factors (individual and center experience). Ilio-femoral artery injuries are typically diagnosed peri-procedurally or early postoperatively, becoming evident in most cases after the device sheath is withdrawn. (Typically, the indwelling sheath provides effective tamponade at the site of injury.) Hemodynamic instability may result in the setting of bleeding from significant vessel rupture, making it imperative to closely monitor hemodynamics at the time of sheath withdrawal. As in this case anecdote, arterial dissection may manifest as lower extremity malperfusion. In more indolent cases, the diagnosis may be made postoperatively via vascular ultrasound, CTA, or peripheral angiography.

Most TAVR centers have adopted measures to decrease the incidence of vascular complications and to recognize them early when they do occur. Careful assessment of pre-procedural CT angiograms for high-risk vascular features (calcification, tortuosity, size) allows for appropriate decision-making about side and location of access and use of surgical cut down or alternate access sites where necessary. Meticulous attention to access technique, including real time ultrasound and fluoroscopy for the initial puncture, decreases the incidence of access site complications. Most centers perform a peripheral angiogram using a small sheath to confirm adequacy of initial access prior to upsizing to the significantly large device sheaths. Following device sheath removal at the end of the case, routine vascular assessment is typically performed using angiography and/or physiologic exam (like PVRs) to assess peripheral flow. In patients with significant calcification, lithotripsy has been shown in some studies to decrease the incidence of vascular complications.

When vascular complications do occur, management depends on the type and severity of injury. Access site hematomas are managed with digital compression and reversal of anticoagulation. Pseudoaneurysms are managed with ultrasound-guided compression or direct thrombin injection, and rarely with open surgical repair. Limited retrograde dissections without meaningful changes in vascular flow are benign and can be managed expectantly. Physiologically significant dissections are managed with endovascular therapies like balloon angioplasty and, if necessary, stenting. In contemporary practices, open surgical repair is rarely necessary. Similarly, endovascular techniques are the mainstay of management in the setting of ilio-femoral vessel rupture. In the setting of bleeding and significant hypovolemic shock, initial efforts are directed toward volume resuscitation and tamponade of the injury either by re-advancing the sheath or by proximal balloon occlusion from the radial artery or contralateral groin. Once relative stability has been achieved, definitive repair can be pursued via placement of covered stents or open surgical repair of long segment or multisite vascular injury.

Bibliography

1. Mangla A, Gupta S. Vascular complications post-transcatheter aortic valve procedures Indian Heart J. 2016;68(5):724–31.
2. Stortecky S, Wenaweser P. Diehm N, Pilgrim T. Huber C, Rosskopf B, Khattab AA, Buellesfeld L, Gloekler S Eberle B. Schmidli J. Carrel T, Meier B, Windecker S. Percutaneous management of vascular complications in patients undergoing transcatheter aortic valve implantation. JACC Cardiovasc Interv. 2012;5(5):515–24.
3. Ruge H, Burri M, Erlebach M, Lange R. Access site related vascular complications with third generation transcatheter heart valve systems. Catheter Cardiovasc Interv. 2020 https://doi.org/10.1002/ccd.29095PMID:32588968DOI:10.1002/ccd.29095.
4. Scarsini R, De Maria GL, Joseph J, Fan L, Cahill TJ, Kotronias RA, Burzotta F, Newton JD, Kharbanda R, Prendergast B, Ribichini F, Banning AP. Impact of complications during transfemoral transcatheter aortic valve replacement: how can they be avoided and managed? J Am Heart Assoc. 2019;8(18):e013801.

Chapter 5
Accidental Arterial Decannulation

Antonia Kreso and Serguei Melnitchouk

Problem

Your 76-year-old neighbor has been complaining of worsening dyspnea on exertion. He has undergone cardiologic workup including echocardiography demonstrating an ejection fraction of 35% and mild mitral regurgitation. Coronary catheterization, showed an 80% proximal LAD lesion, 90% ostial OM2 lesion, and a mid-RCA lesion. Of course, he wants you to do his operation!

You proceed to the operating room where the patient is cooled to 34 °C. The procedure goes smoothly, from initiating bypass to finding good targets. After completing the proximal and distal anastomoses, you begin warming the patient and remove the aortic cross-clamp. The case has gone extrem ely well up to this point. It looks like you're going to make your afternoon meetings with time to spare for lunch. As you begin to place the V-wires, the pacing cable is passed over to anesthesia. Suddenly, there is a sharp pull on the drape, and you are shocked to see (and hear!) a stream of red blood gushing audibly from the patient's aortic cannulation site out of the field. You have never experienced an accidental aortic decannulation and now you have a geyser of crimson blood nearly hitting the OR ceiling! Your sense of calm at the conclusion of a technically flawless operation is now replaced with a rush of adrenalin as you instantly consider your options.

A. Kreso · S. Melnitchouk (✉)
Department of Surgery, Massachusetts General Hospital, Boston, MA, USA
e-mail: Smelnitchouk@mgh.harvard.edu

A. Kreso
e-mail: akreso@mgh.harvard.edu

© The Author(s), under exclusive license to Springer Nature Switzerland AG 2022   17
T. M. Sundt et al. (eds.), *Near Misses in Cardiac Surgery*,
https://doi.org/10.1007/978-3-030-92750-9_5

Solution

The aortic cannula has come out of the patient while on bypass after the cross-clamp has been removed, but before the heart has started beating. Thinking quickly, you grab the aortic cannula in one hand while holding your index finger over the aortotomy site. You ask the perfusionist to stop the pump and shut off the vents but to keep the field suckers going. To prevent air from entering the aorta, you ask anesthesia to place the patient in Trendelenburg position. Then you ask the perfusion team to maintain volume in the heart via the venous cannula in a retrograde fashion, thus filling the heart with residual volume from the venous reservoir. Your assistant then helps you release the snares around the cannulation site to help evacuate air. Next you apply gentle internal cardiac massage. The flaccid aorta begins to fill with the added volume. This allows you to place the cannula into the previous cannulation site. After de-airing the cannula, you reconnect it to the arterial tubing of the circuit and instruct the perfusion team to restart the pump. Placing another purse-string stitch around the cannulation site when the heart starts beating and the patient is stable, you wean off bypass. Examination of the aorta via transesophageal echocardiogram shows no injury to the aortic wall. The patient recovers uneventfully and is discharged on post-operative day five.

Discussion

The approach to managing loss of the arterial cannula during a cardiopulmonary bypass run depends on when the aortic decannulation occurs. If the cannula comes out after the cross-clamp is off and the patient is warm with a beating heart, you can simply attempt to support the patient off bypass. To return volume to the heart, you can ask the perfusion team to perform retrograde transfusion via the venous cannula. Alternatively, the arterial cannula can be inserted into the right atrium for quick return of volume to the patient.

A different scenario is presented if the patient is still cool, and the heart is not beating. Preventing air from entering the aorta is the priority here and the patient should be placed in Trendelenburg position as early as possible. If the cannula falls out while the cross clamp is still on, you need to re-cannulate expeditiously. The cannulation site can be snared with the previously placed stitches. Practical tips for re-cannulating include using the previously placed cannulation site, if possible. However, if this poses a difficulty, the cannula should not be forced into the aorta to avoid a dissection. Instead, the previously placed snares should be tightened to avoid bleeding until a new site is cannulated. It is important to meticulously minimize the risk of air embolus while replacing the cannula. Methods to minimize air include placing the patient in Trendelenburg position and turning off vents to maintain volume in the heart.

Lagniappe (Accidental Arterial Decannulation, *Heart Beating*)

It was a long case. The patient, who was undergoing valve replacement/repair, had prior bypass grafts and there was concern that the innominate vein may be adherent to the back of the sternum. The patient was placed on bypass before opening the chest. This was uneventful and the internal thoracic artery was easily controlled leaving the heart well preserved. Although the procedure was technically difficult, you succeeded in placing the aortic valve and repairing both the mitral and tricuspid valves via an extended superior trans-septal incision. Anticipating a long cross-clamp time, the patient had been cooled to 28 °C for systemic perfusion.

After closing the left atrium, you remove the aortic cross-clamp before seating the tricuspid annuloplasty ring. As you are closing the right atrium, you glance up at the monitor and see that the patient's body temperature is still at 32 °C. Breathing a sigh of relief when the heart starts beating with a narrow complex, you send your assistant on break. The circulating nurse brings a stool for you to sit on as you wait for your assistant to return. Suddenly, the chest fills with bright red blood. Somehow the aortic cannula has become dislodged, and the patient has been decannulated! Your immediate thought is to push the cannula back in, but you can't see the aorta for all the blood.

This is a rare but potentially catastrophic problem. The first step towards a solution here is to gain control of the aortic cannula. Short-handed without an assistant, you ask the staff to STAT page your assistant back to the OR. In the meantime, you manage to free the cannula from the purse-string tourniquets. You ask the perfusion team to stop the arterial flow to the arterial cannula and to leave volume in the patient. You cover the hole over the aorta with your finger and suction the field, revealing the aorta to be partially flaccid. Fortunately, the heart is beating even though the patient is not yet fully warmed. You ask the anesthesia team to ventilate. The patient can do the work for you with a beating heart and ventilating lungs. This gives you time to think while you wait for your assistant to return from break. Upon his/her return, you ask the assistant to snare the aortotomy with the previously placed purse strings. This controls the bleeding from the aorta. You then re-cannulate the aorta at a new location, resume bypass, and finish warming the patient.

Bibliography

1. Kurusz M, Wheeldon DR. Risk containment during cardiopulmonary bypass. Semin Thorac Cardiovasc Surg. 1990;2(4):400–9.

Chapter 6
CABG After MI

Asishana Osho and Nathaniel B. Langer

Problem

You are headed to your car on a Friday evening when your beeper goes off: "STAT. Call now. Cath lab." As you briskly walk back to the hospital, you call the lab and are informed that a 71-year-old male with type 2 diabetes and hypertension was admitted an hour and 10 min ago with severe chest pain, rising troponins, and a new ST-elevation myocardial infarction (STEMI). A prompt diagnostic angiogram demonstrated significant atherosclerosis involving the right coronary artery (RCA) and the mid-left anterior descending artery (LAD). During PCI with stenting of the mid-LAD lesion, the cardiologist noticed extravasation of contrast into the pericardium. Despite placement of a covered stent, the patient became hypotensive, and a pigtail catheter placed in the pericardium drained 400 cc of fresh blood. The patient is hemodynamically stable but is incompletely revascularized, and the cardiologist asks you to take him to the OR immediately. As you ponder this request for an emergent bypass operation, you remember your program director teaching you at several didactic sessions that there is "rarely ever an indication for an emergent CABG." Might you have stumbled upon one of those rare situations? On your way out the door you ask the cardiologists to insert an intra-aortic balloon pump to help you through what you anticipate to be stormy sailing for the next few days.

A. Osho · N. B. Langer (✉)
Department of Surgery, Massachusetts General Hospital, Boston, MA, USA
e-mail: Nlanger@partners.org

A. Osho
e-mail: Asishana.osho@mgh.harvard.edu

© The Author(s), under exclusive license to Springer Nature Switzerland AG 2022   21
T. M. Sundt et al. (eds.), *Near Misses in Cardiac Surgery*,
https://doi.org/10.1007/978-3-030-92750-9_6

Solution

On arrival to the cath lab, you notice the patient moaning on the table, and he tells you that he is still having chest pain. It quickly becomes clear that the team doesn't feel it is safe to continue with PCI, so you call your senior colleague to discuss the case. She agrees that you do in fact have to trade in your Friday night plans with your husband for a date in the operating room. You are delighted to learn that the patient has no evidence of end-organ dysfunction and has not yet received the clopidogrel that had just been ordered—maybe things will be ok after all! Your operating room team mobilizes quickly and an hour later you are making the skin incision. You proceed to perform a three-vessel coronary artery bypass with a left internal mammary artery graft to the LAD and reverse saphenous vein grafts to an early diagonal branch off the LAD and the posterior descending artery (PDA). There is a small hematoma around the area of perforation, but it has been well sealed by the covered stent. The patient separates from cardiopulmonary bypass with robust ventricular function and is discharged home a week later.

Discussion

For patients presenting with new acute coronary syndromes, timely triage into the appropriate category (Category 1: STEMI vs. Category 2: NSTEMI/Unstable Angina) is critical to successful management. For patients with STEMI, immediate reperfusion is the standard of care, with PCI being the most common method for practical reasons. In contemporary practice, CABG has a somewhat limited role, with emergency bypass being indicated for patients who are unable to successfully undergo PCI but have persistent significant ischemia (hemodynamic instability and/or persistent angina) and coronary anatomy that is appropriate for CABG. Certain patterns of coronary obstruction like severe left main disease, severe triple vessel disease, or severe left main equivalents (severe disease involving the proximal LAD and proximal left circumflex) have traditionally been considered surgical disease, although PCI is sometimes performed in these cases, especially when the Syntax score is low. Additionally, patients with post-infarction ventricular septal defects, papillary muscle rupture, or other mechanical complications of myocardial infarction are often better served with immediate surgery for mechanical issues and concurrent revascularization via CABG.

  There are some data suggesting increased mortality for STEMI patients who receive CABG within 24 h of infarction. Authors of these studies recommend waiting at least 3 days post-infarct to perform CABG, postulating that early revascularization with CABG can lead to reperfusion injury manifested as hemorrhagic infarction, extension of myocardial loss, and further scar formation. However, these data are inconsistent, and current guidelines recommend emergency surgery if indicated, regardless of the time elapsed since infarction. In STEMI patients with indications for emergency CABG, clinical drivers of operative timing include evidence of end organ damage and use of anti-platelet therapy. In patients with end organ dysfunction, mechanical circulatory support may be employed to allow for organ recovery prior to surgery. Guidelines recommend waiting at least 24 h before proceeding with CABG for patients who received clopidogrel or ticagrelor (2–4 h for eptifibatide or tirofiban).

In patients with non-ST elevation acute coronary syndromes (NSTE-ACS) including unstable angina and NSTEMI, investigation and revascularization is pursued in a less urgent fashion provided the patient does not have refractory angina, heart failure, or evidence of electrical or hemodynamic instability. If these features are present, triage follows the same pathways outlined above. Guidelines recommend revascularization as soon as possible following infarction for stable NSTE-ACS patients. However, appropriate clinical delays are encouraged prior to CABG in patients who have received platelet inhibitors (clopidogrel 5 days, prasugrel 7 days, abciximab 12 h). Choice of CABG vs. PCI in stable NSTE-ACS patients is determined by comorbidities and anatomy, with CABG being the preference in patients with diabetes, decreased ejection fraction, or any of the specific anatomic features listed above.

Bibliography

1. Yerokun BA, Williams JB, Gaca J, Smith PK, Roe MT. Indications, algorithms, and outcomes for coronary artery bypass surgery in patients with acute coronary syndromes. Coron Artery Dis. 2016;27(4):319–26. https://doi.org/10.1097/MCA.0000000000000364.
2. Pt O, Fg K, Dd A, et al. 2013 ACCF/AHA guideline for the management of ST-elevation myocardial infarction: executive summary: a report of the American College of Cardiology Foundation/American Heart Association Task Force on practice guidelines. Catheter Cardiovasc Interv. 2013;82(1):E1–27. https://doi.org/10.1002/ccd.24776.
3. Lee DC, Oz MC, Weinberg AD, Lin SX, Ting W. Optimal timing of revascularization: transmural versus nontransmural acute myocardial infarction. Ann Thorac Surg. 2001;71 (4):1198–204. https://doi.org/10.1016/S0003-4975(01)02425-0.
4. Amsterdam EA, Wenger NK, Brindis RG, et al. 2014 AHA/ACC Guideline for the management of patients with non-ST-elevation acute coronary syndromes: executive summary: a report of the American college of cardiology/American Heart Association Task Force on practice guidelines. Circulation. 2014;130(25):2354–94. https://doi.org/10.1161/CIR. 0000000000000133.

Chapter 7
Air in the Circuit

Antonia Kreso and Serguei Melnitchouk

Problem

A 75-year-old female presents to your office for evaluation of worsening mitral regurgitation. Her medical history is notable for recent new onset paroxysmal atrial fibrillation. Transthoracic echocardiogram shows an ejection fraction of 65% and severe mitral regurgitation in the setting of A2/A3 segment prolapse with a posteriorly directed jet. Coronary catheterization shows normal coronaries. You recommend mitral valve repair, left atrial appendage amputation, and Maze procedure.

On the day of surgery, you place a central aortic cannula and bicaval venous cannulas. After going on bypass, you place a cross clamp and arrest the heart using antegrade cold blood cardioplegia. You open the left atrium and place a floppy sucker into the left superior pulmonary vein to keep the atrium dry despite residual pulmonary venous return. You amputate the left atrial appendage and perform the left-sided Maze procedure. You then try to expose the mitral valve but notice you are unable to get the field dry of blood as the floppy sucker is not able to handle the pulmonary venous return. After several attempts to fiddle with the floppy sucker, you give up and cut off the protective air filter on that particular vent line to potentially achieve better suction. Finally, you can see the valve well and complete the mitral valve repair by performing a resectional butterfly technique and reinforcing the annulus with a ring. You close the left atriotomy while leaving the floppy sucker in place.

To de-air the system, you place the patient in Trendelenburg position, ask the anesthesiologist to give breaths, and ask the perfusion team to leave volume in and

A. Kreso · S. Melnitchouk (✉)
Division of Cardiac Surgery, Massachusetts General Hospital, 55 Fruit St., Boston, MA 02114, USA
e-mail: smelnitchouk@mgh.harvard.edu

A. Kreso
e-mail: AKreso@mgh.harvard.edu

© The Author(s), under exclusive license to Springer Nature Switzerland AG 2022
T. M. Sundt et al. (eds.), *Near Misses in Cardiac Surgery*,
https://doi.org/10.1007/978-3-030-92750-9_7

turn on the root suction. Once you have de-aired, you remove the aortic cross-clamp and ask for the table to be leveled. Your eye catches a frightening sight, the presence of air in the floppy sucker that is supposed to be acting as a vent! You cannot believe your eyes, but it is true, and you confirm gas bubbles in the root vent. You see a large amount of air go up the aorta and are certain that air has gone to the cerebral circulation.

Solution

Air must have been introduced into the left side of the heart through the floppy sucker, which you have used as a suction with the air filter cut off. Flow on this sucker must have been accidently reversed. You immediately ask the perfusionist to stop flow through the floppy sucker and to completely stop the pump. You instruct anesthesia to place the patient in steep Trendelenburg position. Then, you ask the perfusionist to ensure that there is suction on the floppy sucker and that no shunt has been left open by accident. They start adding vacuum to the floppy sucker and the root vent. You see air being evacuated via the root vent and the floppy sucker. You loosen the purse strings at the aortic cannulation site and actually take the cannula out. You connect the arterial line to the SVC cannula, snare it, clamp the IVC cannula, and ask perfusion to run 300 mL/min of flow through the SVC cannula for retrograde brain perfusion. You begin to see bubbles through the hole in the ascending aorta and also being removed by the aortic root vent. After two minutes, when no further bubbles are noted, you recannulate the aorta, de-air the cannula, reconnect the circuit, and reinstitute cardiopulmonary bypass. You proceed with taking out the LV vent and decannulating in standard fashion. The patient is weaned from cardiopulmonary bypass and transferred to the ICU. She experiences transient ST changes in the RCA distribution that resolve with time. You keep the patient in deep anesthesia postoperatively for two days and the patient receives steroids and barbiturates for cerebral protection. The patient is discharged neurologically intact. You are now in agreement with your mentor: "I hate air. Wish we didn't have to breathe it."

Discussion

While it is rare to have air embolisms with today's cardiopulmonary bypass circuits, it is a potentially disastrous situation when it does happen. Causes can include erroneous flow through a shunt or reversal of flow through a suction line that does not have a protective air filter. If the level of the venous reservoir has gone too low and the alarms are malfunctioning, air can be pumped into the arterial line back into the patient. Irrespective of cause, the management of an air embolism requires rapid, coordinated teamwork by the perfusionist, the anesthesiologist, and the surgeon. The mechanism and extent of air introduced into the left side of the heart will dictate the precise intervention.

For perfusion, if air is introduced through the arterial cannula owing to low venous reservoir volume or a shunt, the cardiopulmonary bypass circuit needs to be discontinued. The arterial and venous lines should be clamped, and the bypass circuit should be de-aired. If there is air in the aortic cannula, the aorta needs to be de-aired by removing the arterial cannula with the patient in Trendelenburg position. Air can be pushed out through the aortic purse string, the aortic cannula de-aired, and then the cannula reinserted back into the patient. Volume in the form of crystalloid can be added to the reservoir by the perfusion team if needed.

Modern cardiopulmonary bypass machines have numerous safety checks and air filters in place to prevent air from returning into the patient. An air filter is also on the LV vent, which in this case was cut off, negating any protection from pumping air. In this case, there was an accidental reversal of flow in the system, where the vent was not suctioning but rather was used to pump volume, or in this case air, into the heart.

From the perspective of anesthesia, the patient must be rapidly placed into steep Trendelenburg position and 100% oxygen administered via the ventilator. Additional agents such as steroids, barbiturates, or mannitol can be administered. The anesthesia team can also support the patient's circulation with vasopressors and inotropes.

From a surgical perspective, air can be aspirated from the aortic root. Retrograde brain perfusion via the SVC (300 mL/min) can be given. Thereafter, cardiopulmonary bypass can be reinstituted, and the patient cooled to 28 °C for brain protection. Also, coronary arteries can be massaged to displace air. After the surgical procedure is completed and de-airing has been achieved in usual fashion, hyperbaric oxygen can be considered postoperatively on an ad-hoc basis.

Bibliography

1. Mills NL, Ochsner JL. Massive air embolism during cardiopulmonary bypass: causes, prevention, and management. J Thorac Cardiovasc Surg. 1980;80:708.
2. Muth CM, Shank ES. Gas embolism. New Engl J Med. 2000;342:476–82.

Chapter 8
EKG Changes after Mitral Repair

Antonia Kreso and Serguei Melnitchouk

Problem

A 65 year-old woman presented to your office with dyspnea on exertion. She had a long-standing history of a murmur and was followed for mitral valve prolapse. Her comorbidities included hypertension, hyperlipidemia, and hypothyroidism. As part of the preoperative workup, she had a transthoracic echocardiogram, which showed P2 prolapse and severe mitral regurgitation with an anteriorly directed jet. EKG-gated CTA showed normal, non-diseased coronary anatomy with a left-dominant system.

The patient is quite concerned about both the cosmetic impact of the procedure and her ability to get back to her favorite past time, ballroom dancing. There is a competition coming up in 3 months and she presses you to get her back on the dance floor as quickly as possible. For the operation, you have suggested a minimally invasive approach via right mini-thoracotomy with femoral cannulation. You are not sure if the patients actually experience less pain from this approach than sternotomy, but it is clear they get back to activity sooner, whether physiologic or psychologic. You enter the left atrium using a trans-atrial approach and find P2 prolapse with ruptured chords. You repair the valve by placing 4 neochords to P2 and reinforce the mitral annulus with a complete ring. After you have de-aired and closed the atriotomy, you start rewarming and take off the cross-clamp. The heart starts regaining a rhythm and as you are checking for hemostasis, your eye catches

A. Kreso · S. Melnitchouk (✉)
Department of Surgery, Massachusetts General Hospital, Boston, MA, USA
e-mail: smelnitchouk@mgh.harvard.edu

A. Kreso
e-mail: akreso@mgh.harvard.edu

© The Author(s), under exclusive license to Springer Nature Switzerland AG 2022
T. M. Sundt et al. (eds.), *Near Misses in Cardiac Surgery*,
https://doi.org/10.1007/978-3-030-92750-9_8

an unwanted sight on the EKG tracing: ST elevations along the lateral leads. The patient becomes hypotensive requiring high dose epinephrine and norepinephrine. As the patient's blood pressure is dropping, yours is rising, knowing that this is going to be a much longer case than you expected.

Solution

While asking the anesthesia team to look at the lateral wall, you go back on bypass using the femoral cannulas. The anesthesia team informs you there is no discreet wall motion abnormality. Despite this, you know the EKG tracing is abnormal in this patient with a left-dominant system. You ask your assistant to harvest a segment of vein. Discouraged, you open the chest via sternotomy and arrest the heart. You find a large OM target, which you bypass using the venous conduit. Once this is done you remove the cross-clamp and come off the bypass without issues. The previously seen ST segment changes on the lateral wall have now resolved. You complete the remainder of the case, and the patient recovers well postoperatively. Aside from an additional incision, the patient's recovery is unremarkable, and she is discharged home on postoperative day 4.

Discussion

The reason for hemodynamic compromise was a left circumflex artery occlusion most likely due to deep stitches while placing the mitral ring. Although easier said than done via a mini-thoracotomy approach, the needle tip should always be oriented toward the ventricle, especially when placing annular stitches near the left trigone and along the base of the P1 scallop. A misplaced stitch can either kink, stenose, or completely occlude the artery [1, 2]. One option to restore blood flow is to take out the ring and replace it with new stitches [3]. This risks further ischemia to the heart and will not guarantee the problem is fixed. The safer option is to restore circulation to the heart by creating a bypass graft if hemodynamically significant changes are seen when weaning off bypass.

Whenever ST changes are seen after cardiac surgery, the differential needs to include air embolism or iatrogenic injury. In the setting of a mitral valve repair or replacement and isolated EKG changes, damage to the coronary artery is the likely culprit. This may be confirmed by examining the lateral wall with intra-operative trans-esophageal echocardiography. However, this may not always show wall motion abnormalities and therefore should not be relied upon to make the definitive diagnosis of malperfusion. Frequently, ST changes are seen along the distribution of the right coronary artery and the usual culprit is air that has traveled into the right coronary circulation during de-airing. However, if ST changes are seen along the distribution of the left circumflex, particularly in a left dominant system during mitral valve surgery, strong suspicion is centered around iatrogenic damage to the left circumflex artery.

It is important to remember that a valve or ring causing traction on the circumflex due to excessive pull can cause delayed myocardial ischemia. Special attention needs to be paid to ensure safety of the circumflex artery. If there is an intra-operative concern, a marginal branch can be bypassed using SVG prior to coming off cardiopulmonary bypass. Assessing the location and flow in the circumflex artery in relation to the annulus can be helpful if done routinely on pre- and post-bypass transesophageal echocardiography.

References

1. Aybek T, Risteski P, Miskovic A, Simon A, Dogan S, Abdel-Rahman U, Moritz A. Seven years' experience with suture annuloplasty for mitral valve repair. J Thorac Cardiovasc Surg. 2006;131(1):99–106.
2. Nakajima H, Ikari Y, Kigawa I, Kitamura T, Hatori M, Tooda E, Tanabe K, Miyairi T, Hara K. Rapid diagnosis and management of intraoperative myocardial infarction during valvular surgery: using intraoperative transesophageal echocardiography followed by emergency coronary artery bypass grafting without coronary angiography. Echocardiography. 2005;22 (10):834–8.
3. Ender J, Selbach M, Borger MA, Krohmer E, Falk V, Kaisers UX, Mohr FW, Mukherjee C. Echocardiographic identification of iatrogenic injury of the circumflex artery during minimally invasive mitral valve repair. Ann Thorac Surg. 2010;89(6):1866–72.

Chapter 9
ECMO as a Bridge

Asishana Osho and Nathaniel B. Langer

Problem

Ms. M is in the emergency department (ED) with a symptomatic pleural effusion. Her CABG went as smoothly as one could have hoped, and she was discharged two weeks ago after an uneventful course. Expecting to perform a bedside thoracentesis and prevent a readmission, you head to the ED after your last clinic patient on Friday afternoon. Your determined march is interrupted in front of ED bay 1 when the ED attending—your former medical school classmate—flags you down and tells you she has someone who might need heart surgery right away! She introduces you to a 52 year-old man who presented to the ED with 5 days of chest pain, shortness of breath, and anuria. He drove himself to the hospital but is now requiring escalating doses of peripheral norepinephrine to maintain his blood pressure. Workup so far is notable for markedly elevated serum lactate, serum creatinine, and liver function tests. His EKG shows inferior ST segment elevations, and a transthoracic echocardiogram demonstrates inferior wall akinesis, severe right ventricular dysfunction, and evidence of flow between the left and right ventricles. The interventional cardiology service has been called and an urgent angiogram is being arranged. You are tempted to defer further management to the cardiology team while you perform the thoracentesis a few rooms down and hopefully avoid another readmission on your report card. However, as you peer into bay 1 at a progressively somnolent and diaphoretic patient, it becomes increasingly clear that without intervention, this patient may not survive to see the cath lab.

A. Osho · N. B. Langer (✉)
Department of Surgery, Massachusetts General Hospital, Boston, MA, USA
e-mail: Nlanger@partners.org

A. Osho
e-mail: Asishana.osho@mgh.harvard.edu

© The Author(s), under exclusive license to Springer Nature Switzerland AG 2022
T. M. Sundt et al. (eds.), *Near Misses in Cardiac Surgery*,
https://doi.org/10.1007/978-3-030-92750-9_9

Solution

After quickly reviewing the rest of the chart, you help the team obtain central access for monitoring and medications. You have the prospicience to place ultrasound-guided femoral arterial and venous sheaths in case 'the patient further deteriorates. The cath lab staff is on the way, and you know they will be here within 30 min—they are proud of their "door-to-balloon" statistics—but the patient's mean arterial pressure is now lingering close to 50 mm Hg despite escalation of multiple vasopressors. You activate the extra-corporeal membrane oxygenation (ECMO) team and obtain additional access for a distal perfusor on the side of the femoral arterial sheath before cannulating the patient for ECMO with a 17 Fr arterial cannula and a 23–25 Fr venous cannula. You take the time in the ED before transport to optimize the patient's flow parameters, after which he is whisked off to the cath lab for a drug eluting stent to an acutely occluded right coronary artery. There is a 60% stenosis in the LAD but the circumflex is free of disease. A left ventriculogram confirms your suspicion of a post-infarct ventricular septal defect (VSD).

You consider taking him directly to the OR for repair but are concerned about his renal and hepatic dysfunction. Instead you support him over the next four days on ECMO. To your relief his perfusion parameters improve significantly, lactate resolves, and liver enzymes trend down just as his renal function improves. By the time you take him to the operating room five days after his initial presentation for coronary artery bypass grafting and repair of his VSD, his creatinine and liver function tests are back to normal, and he has demonstrated significant myocardial recovery. The operation is completed uneventfully, although you cautiously return to the ICU on ECMO to give his right heart more time to bounce back. Thankfully, his myocardial recovery continues, and he is decannulated from ECMO two days later. He is discharged from the hospital three weeks after the initial presentation.

Discussion

Patients with cardiogenic shock and indications for cardiac interventions represent a challenging population that continues to have high mortality despite technological improvements. This is best demonstrated in the management of patients with acute myocardial ischemia, where mortality is $\sim 5\%$ in the absence of cardiogenic shock versus upwards of 45% in patients with cardiogenic shock. This mortality difference is driven by variations in the severity of cardiac disease to some degree, but also by the debilitating effects of multi-organ failure when present preoperatively. Renal failure seldom improves with a pump run! This is further supported by data highlighting an association between acute kidney or liver injury and increased mortality following cardiac surgery.

In patients with indications for cardiac surgery, such as post-infarct VSD or papillary muscle rupture, the technological improvements in veno-arterial (VA) ECMO technology are making pre-intervention support for end organ recovery an increasingly appealing option. When properly managed, VA-ECMO often permits significant decreases in inotrope requirements, theoretically promoting recovery of vulnerable myocytes in the border zone and reducing infarct size. This may be of particular value in the specific setting of inferior posterior infarct VSD, where associated right ventricular infarction and resultant failure are largely accountable for the higher mortality rate observed as compared with anterior VSD. Importantly, while ECMO provides circulatory support, it is not adequate therapy in patients with untreated ischemic cardiac disease. In these patients, ECMO support does not obviate the need for rapid coronary interrogation and potentially percutaneous intervention where indicated. Mechanical complications of myocardial infarction are most commonly observed in patients with single-vessel coronary artery disease where there has been insufficient time for the development of collateral circulation and, accordingly, the infarct territory is densely injured. ECMO may also be of value in the setting of massive pulmonary embolus with hemodynamic collapse or other unspecified causes of cardiac arrest for "extracorporeal CPR" or "ECPR".

ECMO for cardiogenic shock is most easily initiated using cannulas in the femoral artery and femoral vein. With this approach, ECMO can be started rapidly with minimal bleeding issues particularly when access is obtained percutaneously. In patients with poor LV ejection, aortic insufficiency, or mitral regurgitation, special attention must be paid to decompression of the left ventricle (LV). ECMO does not unload the LV but actually increases afterload, and distention on ECMO can lead to further myocyte damage and pulmonary edema. In cases where LV distention persists despite optimization of volume and LV loading conditions, direct decompression of the LV can be performed using percutaneous or surgical techniques with axial flow pumps placed across the aortic valve or vents connected to the circuit. ECMO can also be established centrally by placing cannulas in the aorta and the right atrium. This approach is associated with higher rates of bleeding complications and has the added disadvantage of disrupting planes in patients who may eventually need surgery. It may, however, be more appropriate in patients at high risk for LV distention as it allows for direct placement of vents which can be connected to the ECMO circuit.

Bibliography

1. Rao P, Khalpey Z, Smith R, Burkhoff D, Kociol RD. Venoarterial extracorporeal membrane oxygenation for cardiogenic shock and cardiac arrest. Circ Heart Fail. 2018;11(9):e004905. https://doi.org/10.1161/CIRCHEARTFAILURE.118.004905.
2. Wallinder A, Pellegrino V, Fraser JF, McGiffin DC. ECMO as a bridge to non-transplant cardiac surgery. J Card Surg. 2017;32(8):514–21. https://doi.org/10.1111/jocs.13172.

3. Sheu JJ, Tsai TH, Lee FY, et al. Early extracorporeal membrane oxygenator-assisted primary percutaneous coronary intervention improved 30-day clinical outcomes in patients with ST-segment elevation myocardial infarction complicated with profound cardiogenic shock. Crit Care Med. 2010;38(9):1810–7. https://doi.org/10.1097/CCM.0b013e3181e8acf7.
4. Kwon J, Lee D. The effectiveness of extracorporeal membrane oxygenation in a patient with post myocardial infarct ventricular septal defect. J Cardiothorac Surg. 2016;11(1):143. https://doi.org/10.1186/s13019-016-0537-5.
5. David TE, Armstrong S. Surgical repair of postinfarction ventricular septal defect by infarct exclusion. Semin Thorac Cardiovasc Surg. 1998;10(2):105–10. https://doi.org/10.1016/s1043-0679(98)70003-6 PMID: 9620457.

Chapter 10
Complications of Transcatheter Aortic Valve Replacement (TAVR)

Asishana Osho and Nathaniel B. Langer

Problem

Another TAVR day has gone well and the only thing standing between you and your drive home is deployment of the valve in an 83 year-old man with severe aortic stenosis. You aren't usually this tired after a day of percutaneous interventions, but you spent much of the previous evening at a mandatory team-based exercise on managing intraoperative emergencies. "Great way to spend an evening," you sarcastically murmur to yourself as the fellow advances the valve first across the aortic arch, then the aortic valve. You re-focus for the deployment process, noting the initiation of pacing, the root angiogram, and the inflation of the balloon. Half-way through deployment, however, there is an abrupt loss of pacing. In an attempt to prevent distal embolization, the operator pushes on the delivery system, and he valve drops into the ventricle.

Solution

You immediately initiate a quick conversation with your interventional cardiology colleagues about potentially retrieving the valve using a wire and a balloon. Remembering points about team mobilization from the session the prior evening, you inform the anesthesiologist about the possibility of open conversion and page your chief resident to assist you. Additionally, you tell the perfusion team what to have available in case of cardiopulmonary bypass and confirm the presence of

A. Osho · N. B. Langer (✉)
Department of Surgery, Massachusetts General Hospital, Boston, MA, USA
e-mail: Nlanger@partners.org

A. Osho
e-mail: Asishana.osho@mgh.harvard.edu

© The Author(s), under exclusive license to Springer Nature Switzerland AG 2022   37
T. M. Sundt et al. (eds.), *Near Misses in Cardiac Surgery*,
https://doi.org/10.1007/978-3-030-92750-9_10

blood products in the room. After a quick assessment of the live fluoroscopy, it is determined that a percutaneous rescue will not be possible in this case. You take a second to do a brief huddle with the entire team and then proceed to open the chest. You quickly cannulate and go on bypass, arrest the heart, and then open the aorta. After resecting the leaflets of the native valve, you manage to retrieve the embolized TAVR valve from just underneath the mitral valve. You perform a surgical aortic valve replacement without any issues. When the case is discussed at the next mortality and morbidity conference, your team commends you for your exemplary leadership, and "for your sins," unanimously recommends that you lead the session on intraoperative emergencies at the next series of team building exercises. What a turn of events!

Discussion

Reported rates of device embolization during TAVR range from 0.1 to 1.1%. Risk of embolization is higher in the setting of valve under-sizing, high valve deployment, failure or early termination of pacing, and incomplete inflation and/or failure to retract the pusher of the delivery system. Anatomic factors like low burden of annular calcification, left ventricular hypertrophy, or protruding mitral prosthesis struts have also been associated with valve embolization. Embolization happens almost exclusively with balloon expandable prostheses, as self-expanding valves are equipped with recapture and repositioning capabilities. Valve embolization can be in the proximal direction—into the ventricle—or distally into the ascending aorta. The immediate clinical consequences are generally quite benign, although hemodynamic instability can occur if there is further obstruction of an already critical left ventricular outflow tract or interaction with the mitral apparatus causing acute severe regurgitation. Fortunately, this complication is generally recognized immediately as deployment is performed using direct, real time fluoroscopy.

There are reports of percutaneous solutions to TAVR embolization, particularly when embolization occurs into the aorta. These cases generally involve placement of a guidewire through the embolized valve which prevents rotation and allows for inflation of a balloon in the aorta, proximal to the valve. The balloon can then be used to pull the valve to a secure, branchless location in the descending aorta where it may be deployed. The valve may then be secured in the open position using an endovascular stent, and studies suggest limited consequence of having a second functioning valve in the descending aorta. TAVR may then be performed at the aortic annulus as initially planned.

TAVR embolization into the ventricle can also be managed with percutaneous approaches if the valve can be retracted sufficiently into the upper left ventricular outflow tract. Reports of such interventions have encouraged the use of a second valve to overlap the first, thus providing additional security. Often however, TAVR embolization into the ventricle requires sternotomy for surgical removal given the increased likelihood of valve rotation and the potential for disruption of left ventricular structures.

Bibliography

1. Moreno-Samos JC, Vidovich MI. Device embolization in transcatheter aortic valve procedures: expect the unexpected. Editorial Comment J Am Coll Cardiol Case Rep. 2019;2:105–11.
2. Vendrik J, van den Boogert TPW, Koch KT, Baan J. Balloon-expandable TAVR prosthesis dislocates into the ascending aorta. Case Report: Clinical Case J Am Coll Cardiol Case Rep. 2019;1(2):101–4.
3. Kim W-K, Schäfer U, Tchetche D, Holger, et al. Incidence and outcome of peri-procedural transcatheter heart valve embolization and migration: the TRAVEL registry (TranscatheteR HeArt Valve EmboLization and Migration). Euro Heart J. 2019;40(38):3156–65. https://doi.org/10.1093/eurheartj/ehz429.
4. Alkhouli M, Sievert H, Rihal CS. Device embolization in structural heart interventions: incidence, outcomes, and retrieval techniques state-of-the-art review. J Am Coll Cardiol Cardiovasc Interv. 2019;12(2):113–26.
5. Dumonteil N, Marcheix B, Grunenwald E, Roncalli J, Massabuau P, Carrié D. Left ventricular embolization of an aortic balloon-expandable bioprosthesis: balloon capture and reimpaction as an alternative to emergent conversion to open-heart surgery images. In Intervention J Am Coll Cardiol Cardiovasc Interv. 2013;6(3):308–10.

Chapter 11
Catastrophic Bleeding from Right Atrium

Andrew C. W. Baldwin and Thoralf M. Sundt

Problem

The case had been tough—an acute dissection in a 42 year-old man with no apparent connective tissue disease but likely poorly controlled hypertension. Although he had never consulted a doctor about his hypertension, his whole family had the condition. Full of the confidence and optimism that accompanies a mid-afternoon dissection, you began with plans for a hemi-arch and valve-sparing root, but the distal anastomosis fell apart and you had to struggle through a brachiocephalic reconstruction beyond the subclavian. To add insult to injury, the aortic valve leaked when you took off the clamp and you had to replace it as well. Exhausted, you made it home in the early hours of the morning only to be STAT paged to the ICU immediately after sitting down with a warm cup of coffee.

The ICU staff tells you that the patient underwent endotracheal suctioning in anticipation of extubation. After a brief coughing spell, dark blood began pouring out from the mediastinal chest tubes. Suspecting it was either the venous cannulation or retrograde cardioplegia site, you quickly change into scrubs while the team mobilizes for the OR. The only room available is in the general surgery wing, and when you arrive it is clear you need to open the chest before a pump can be set up. After a quick prep and drape with a nameless general surgery intern (the only available assistant), you remove the wires, open the chest, and your suspicion is confirmed. The retrograde cardioplegia cannulation site has blown out. You put

A. C. W. Baldwin
Division of Cardiac Surgery, Straub Medical Center, Honolulu, HI, USA
e-mail: Andrew.Baldwin@hphmg.org

T. M. Sundt (✉)
Division of Cardiac Surgery, Massachusetts General Hospital, Boston, MA, USA
e-mail: tsundt@mgh.harvard.edu

© The Author(s), under exclusive license to Springer Nature Switzerland AG 2022   41
T. M. Sundt et al. (eds.), *Near Misses in Cardiac Surgery*,
https://doi.org/10.1007/978-3-030-92750-9_11

your finger over the hole while the anesthesiologists resuscitate the patient and the perfusionists prime the pump in a cramped room. There is no experienced help available, and you stare at your finger in the dyke wondering what you're going to do next.

Solution

Although the bleeding seems torrential when you take your finger off the hole, how big can it really be? You ask the scrub to load a backhanded 3-0 Prolene on an SH needle, confident you can get this under control. You place a figure-of-eight suture, passing the needle under your own finger, and ask the yet unidentified intern to cover the hole while you tie down the suture. Frustratingly, the atrium is so thin that what was a relatively small hole seconds ago is now the size of a dime. Seeking easy stress relief, you chide the still innominate intern for his ungraceful assistance. Taking a deep breath, you break down the problem and realize the priority now is stopping the bleeding, not necessarily closing the hole.

You quickly run through your options. You consider going on bypass to decompress the atrium, but central cannulation would be challenging given your graft repair. Femoral arterial cannulation is unappealing in the setting of a dissection. Instead, you call for a Foley catheter with a 10 cc balloon and ask the scrub to clamp the central channel. You slip the catheter into the hole under your finger and blow up the balloon in the atrium. Pulling the balloon gently back it obstructs the hole. Now you've got time to think, to get your team in place, and to execute a plan.

Given the fragility of the right atrium, you carefully place a pledgeted purse string in the atrium wide of the Foley balloon using a small needle on a 4-0 stitch, deflate the balloon, and extract the Foley as you tie down the suture. You thank the intern for his help and ask him to transport your patient back to the unit while you search for a new cup of coffee.

Discussion

Catastrophic bleeding from an atrial source occurs rarely, so the surgeon needs to be prepared with an algorithm in mind if it does. The source may be the atrial purse string itself or, as in this instance, the site of the retrograde cardioplegia cannula. For this reason, many surgeons routinely reinforce all cannulation sites and some even routinely use pledgeted sutures for particularly susceptible sites such as the retrograde cardioplegia cannulation which often passes through a very thin portion of the atrium. You failed to do so in this case, no doubt because you were exhausted by the lengthy case you just experienced. This is when it is most critically important to be aware of your own mental condition and seek the opinions of the team around you who may in fact be thinking more sharply than are you. It is critically important that you be aware of your own mental reserve. In a state like this it may be prudent as a rule to set your mental default to "yes" and not "no" for suggestions made by others who may have just scrubbed in on the case. The key to resilience is teamwork and the key to teamwork is open communication including receptivity to suggestions.

When bleeding such as this is venous in nature, you may well have time to move the patient from the ICU to the OR. While catastrophic arterial bleeding can be rapidly fatal due to tamponade and begs for immediate chest exploration in the ICU, the mode of exit secondary to venous bleeding is exsanguination, so there is an opportunity to transfuse the patient and transfer to the OR as the rate of bleeding will slow as the CVP drops and the pressure in the pericardial space rises. Clamping the chest tubes may therefore be a prudent step sufficient to slow the bleeding before hemodynamic collapse. Certainly, the options for repair, including access to a pump, are better in the OR, so when possible, it makes sense to resuscitate the patient on the floor and then transfer to the OR.

Once confronted with this bleeding source, attempting to simply place a figure-of-eight suture is tempting and may be successful, but the volume of bleeding, even if venous in nature, can be so overwhelming that what seems an easy task rapidly becomes impossible, especially without adequate assistance. It is more prudent to get the bleeding under control, pause until you have your team available, and then attack the problem in a measured and coherent way.

Bibliography

1. Dunning J, Nandi J, Ariffin S, Jerstice J, Danitsch D, Levine A. The cardiac surgery advanced life support course (CALS): delivering significant improvements in emergency cardiothoracic care. Ann Thorac Surg. 2006;81(5):1767–72.
2. Charalambous CP, Zipitis CS, Keenan DJ. Chest reexploration in the intensive care unit after cardiac surgery: a safe alternative to returning to the operating theater. Ann Thorac Surg. 2006;81:191–4.
3. Whelehan DF, McCarrick CA, Ridgway PF. A systematic review of sleep deprivation and technical skill in surgery. Surgeon. 2020;18:375–84.
4. Wilson SM, Au FC. In extremis use of a Foley catheter in a cardiac stab wound. J Trauma. 1986;26:400–2.
5. Feliciano DV, Burch JM, Mattox KL, Bitondo CG, Fields G. Balloon catheter tamponade in cardiovascular wounds. Am J Surg. 1990;160(6):583–7.

Chapter 12
Hypoxia on Bypass

Antonia Kreso and Serguei Melnitchouk

Problem

You have recognized that the field of cardiac surgery is increasingly subspecialized and that in order to have an exemplary clinical practice, you must strive to focus your efforts and energies to become a leader in your selected sub-specialty. You have chosen the domain of valvular heart disease and structural interventions including mitral valve repair. In the current era, a less than 95% repair rate for degenerative disease involving the posterior mitral leaflet is unacceptable. With successful repair first and foremost in your mind you head to the operating room to care for a 61 year-old woman with hypertension and a history of migraines who presented with shortness of breath on exertion and was found to have severe mitral regurgitation. Preoperative workup included an echocardiogram that showed an ejection fraction of 75%, normal aortic valve, mild tricuspid valve regurgitation, and a pliable mitral valve with isolated posterior leaflet prolapse. We plan to perform the procedure via a right mini-thoracotomy.

You cannulate the femoral vessels for bypass and place an antegrade cardioplegia cannula in the ascending aorta. After going on bypass without issues, you cross clamp the aorta and give antegrade cardioplegia with a quick arrest of the heart. All appears to be going well with the perfusionist reporting full bypass flows at the target level. The ventilator has been turned off and you are taking your seat at the tableside, opening the pericardium. Just as you begin dissecting the inter-atrial groove to access the left atrium for mitral valve repair the anesthesia team informs you the oxygen saturation is 88% and has been gradually dropping ever since going on bypass. You experience that uncomfortable feeling having to refocus your

A. Kreso · S. Melnitchouk (✉)
Department of Surgery, Massachusetts General Hospital, Boston, MA, USA
e-mail: Smelnitchouk@mgh.harvard.edu

A. Kreso
e-mail: akreso@mgh.harvard.edu

© The Author(s), under exclusive license to Springer Nature Switzerland AG 2022
T. M. Sundt et al. (eds.), *Near Misses in Cardiac Surgery*,
https://doi.org/10.1007/978-3-030-92750-9_12

mental energy from the technical aspects of successful repair to troubleshooting a perfusion problem. Just as you tell yourself that perhaps the problem will go away, the anesthesia team complains that the oxygen saturation has dropped to 84%. How can this be? The perfusion team tells you they are giving 100% FiO2 and have not had any issues with pump flow.

Solution

Taking a deep breath you acknowledge that the most immediate problem to be solved is the patient's hypoxia, not the mitral regurgitation. Trying to achieve full situational awareness you glance over at the groin and are struck by the fact that the blood in both circuit lines has a similar color. You turn to the perfusion team because you know the oxygenation function of the cardiopulmonary bypass system is not performing as it should. The first step in this scenario is to confirm the integrity of all the connections, starting with the gas supply to the oxygenator. Here you discover that the line connecting the oxygenator to the oxygen supply from the wall has been disconnected, likely when the circuit was moved closer to the operative field to pass the lines. The perfusion team quickly reconnects the oxygen line and you see a gradual change in color of the arterial cannula. The oxygen saturations return to 100%. Relieved you now aim to get your head back into the technical aspects of successful mitral repair. It turns out this was a relatively simple problem to solve, but disruptions to the flow of an operation such as this are unsettling and can contribute to subsequent errors and accidents. Recognizing this you take a moment to pause, refocus, and carefully proceed asking anyone in the operating room who sees you beginning to do something foolish to speak up. You know you are now in a vulnerable state and you will take all the help you can get. Fortunately, the remainder of the case is finished without issues and the repair goes well. The patient does well postoperatively.

Discussion

Oxygenation problems can be grouped into two categories. Acute loss of oxygen delivery to the patient's venous blood is evident by a change in the color of the arterial line to dark blood. If this happens, the first step is to provide oxygen to the patient. The patient's lungs should be ventilated to facilitate oxygen delivery if the heart is beating and blood is flowing through the lungs. Next, the oxygen delivery system on the cardiopulmonary bypass machine needs to be interrogated. This can be achieved by checking the gas supply connection. If it is disconnected, as in this case, the problem can be quickly resolved by simply reconnecting the oxygen tubing line. However, if the connection is functional, the priority should be to connect the oxygenator to a fresh oxygen source. For this, a new oxygen tank should be brought into the room and directly connected to the oxygenator. If this does not solve the problem, the oxygenator itself is not functioning correctly.

Intrinsic oxygenator failure is usually not an acute scenario but presents once the patient has been on bypass for some time. Typical findings will be a decrease in the PaO_2 and an increase of the PCO_2. The perfusion team will correct these values by increasing the FiO_2 and sweep. However, if this does not fix the problem, the oxygenator should be exchanged. Oxygenator failure can occur due to blockages of the micropores, which can be caused by protein leakage, high platelet counts, or blood clots.

Exchanging an oxygenator can be a challenging scenario if the patient is on full cardiopulmonary bypass with the cross clamp on. If the patient's heart is pumping and the patient is either going on or just coming off bypass, the patient can be supported by ventilating the lungs and weaning from bypass, even if not yet fully rewarmed. If such situation arises during the cross-clamp time, one can also sometimes remove the cross clamp and initiate an internal heart massage. Obviously, this maneuver can only be done safely when no cardiac chamber is open. Major trouble arises if this happens in the setting of an open-heart chamber, such as with an aortic valve that has just been debrided. For this reason, it is critical to verify with the team whether the bypass circuit is functioning correctly before taking an irreversible (or difficult to reverse) step. These "single point vulnerabilities" or "single point failures" are a focus of attention in the nuclear power industry and call for particular awareness and mental focus.

To exchange an oxygenator, another perfusionist must be in the room to help. A new oxygenator is brought into the room and the ancillary lines are changed (including the heat exchanger and the temperature sensor). Once the ancillary lines have been connected, the perfusionist needs to be able to quickly exchange the oxygenator. This is achieved by first clamping the arterial and venous lines to the patient. Next the inflow, outflow, cardioplegia system, and re-circulation line need to be clamped to the oxygenator. This will allow you to put on a new oxygenator and then re-connect the lines. Next, the system must be de-aired. To safely de-air the system, the bridge between the venous and arterial lines needs to unclamped (this bridge, or shunt, is kept clamped during a CPB run), while clamping the actual lines to the patient. This way, the patient is protected from accidental air entrainment and the perfusion team can prime the new oxygenator. Once the system is well deaired, the tubing clamps to the patient can be removed and cardiopulmonary bypass can be resumed.

Lagniappe (Oxygenator Failure, Oxygenator Needs to Be Replaced)

Problem

You have just gotten through your first year of practice, likely the most stressful year of your professional life. You have started to build a referral base and are delighted to see a referral from one of the private practice groups that typically refer only to the chief, who happens to be out of town. The patient is a 65 year-old female with severe symptomatic aortic stenosis secondary to a bicuspid aortic valve. She has no coronary artery disease, and you are looking forward to a straightforward aortic valve replacement. You cannulate the aorta, place a dual stage venous cannula, and go on bypass, cooling to 34 °C. You are just about to apply the cross-clamp when your pager goes off. Wisely, you decide that it is better to see if there is an urgent issue before cross-clamping the aorta. The circulating nurse answers the page and informs you that the ICU is wondering whether one of your patients can be sent to the stepdown unit. A little irritated by this distraction, you answer "Yes" and turn your attention back to the operation. As you are about to apply the cross-clamp, you realize that the blood in the arterial cannula looks surprisingly dark. You ask the perfusionist if the oxygenator is functioning properly. Horrified, they reply "No!"

Solution

You are now faced with a patient on the cardiopulmonary bypass machine without oxygenation. Luckily the patient still has two functional lungs! The main principle in managing oxygenator failure in such a situation is to come off cardiopulmonary bypass, let the patient oxygenate by turning on the ventilator, and then turn your attention to fixing the oxygenator issue without time pressure.

You ask the anesthesia team to ventilate the patient while the perfusion team starts to troubleshoot the cause of the oxygenator failure. Since the patient has a perfusing rhythm and you are not cross clamped, you ask the perfusionist to come off bypass until the perfusionist can call for help and troubleshoot the circuit. They discover this is not a matter of a disconnection but of the oxygenator itself which needs to be changed out. A second perfusionist arrives with a new oxygenator. The tubing toward the patient is clamped, the oxygenator is replaced, and the system is deaired. This takes several minutes even with two experienced perfusionists in the room.

You are thankful that the patient's heart is beating, knowing that if it was not, you would have been forced to perform open cardiac massage until the oxygenator could be changed. A good checkpoint is to always confirm with the perfusionist regarding the function of their pump prior to committing to an irreversible (or difficult to reverse) action, such as stopping the heart. In this case, the ICU's interruption, despite your irritation, has helped to avoid a potentially disastrous problem.

Bibliography

1. Webb DP, Deegan RJ, Greelish JP, Byrne JG. Oxygenation failure during cardiopulmonary bypass prompts new safety algorithm and training initiative. J Extra Corpor Technol. 2007;39 (3):188–91.
2. Soo A, et al. Successful management of membrane oxygenator failure during cardiopulmonary bypass—the importance of safety algorithm and simulation drills. J Extra Corpor Technol. 2012;44(2):78–80.
3. de Leval MR, Carthey J, Wright DJ, Farewell VT, Reason JT. Human factors and cardiac surgery: a multicenter study. J Thorac Cardiovasc Surg. 2000;119(4 Pt 1):661–72. https://doi. org/10.1016/S0022-5223(00)70006-7 PMID: 10733754.
4. Wiegmann DA, ElBardissi AW, Dearani JA, Daly RC, Sundt TM 3rd. Disruptions in surgical flow and their relationship to surgical errors: an exploratory investigation. Surgery. 2007;142 (5):658–65. https://doi.org/10.1016/j.surg.2007.07.034 PMID: 17981185.

Chapter 13
Challenges in Myocardial Protection

Brittany Potz and George Tolis

Problem

You are pleased to have established a reputation in aortic root surgery, although with it come some imposing challenges. You have just been referred a case involving a 68 year-old man who underwent homograft aortic valve replacement 15 years ago when enthusiasm for the long-term durability of these homografts was high. Sadly, this optimism has proved to be misplaced, and you are now seeing patients come back with calcified roots and severely regurgitant valves. Furthermore, this gentleman also had a LITA placed to his LAD which is now totally occluded proximally but beautifully supplied by the graft. The new resident on your service is excited to scrub on this "great case" and is full of questions about myocardial protection, the subject of last week's didactic presentation.

In the operating room you accomplish an uneventful re-entry. The adhesions are thankfully scant as you separate the right atrium from the pericardium from IVC to SVC and identify the native aorta above the homograft. The homograft is as hard as a rock (of calcium) but there is a neck of ascending aorta adequate for cannulation and clamping. You find the LIMA graft outside the pericardium medial to the left lung and control it with a silastic tape. You administer heparin and cannulate the ascending aorta, placing a 2-stage venous return cannula via the right atrial appendage. Despite multiple attempts to place a retrograde cannula through the right atrium, it is impossible to direct the cannula through the coronary sinus. You know that antegrade cardioplegia will be inadequate for induction of diastolic arrest since there is wide open aortic insufficiency. Moreover, ostial cardioplegia is

B. Potz
Department of Surgery, Massachusetts General Hospital, Boston, MA, USA
e-mail: bpotz@mgh.harvard.edu

G. Tolis (✉)
Department of Surgery, Brigham and Women's Hospital, Boston, MA, USA
e-mail: gtolis@partners.org

© The Author(s), under exclusive license to Springer Nature Switzerland AG 2022
T. M. Sundt et al. (eds.), *Near Misses in Cardiac Surgery*,
https://doi.org/10.1007/978-3-030-92750-9_13

51

unlikely to protect the anterior wall well since the native LAD is entirely perfused by the beautifully mature LIMA graft.

What are your options?

Solution

You reason that the delivery of retrograde cardioplegia is critical. You simply must get access to the inside of the right atrium to insert the cannula under direct vision. Reluctantly, you remove the 2-stage cannula and replace it with SVC and IVC cannulae. After commencing bypass and securing caval tapes, you place a bulldog on the LITA and cross clamp the aorta prior to opening the right atrium in case there is an undiagnosed PFO (as happens all too often). You insert the retrograde catheter into the coronary sinus and begin delivering cardioplegia. With your assistant ensuring appropriate position, you place a purse-string suture and tourniquet around the ostium ensuring adequate delivery and relax. A long operation ahead, but the heart will be protected.

Discussion

Adequate myocardial protection is of utmost importance in any open-heart operation involving cross clamping and diastolic arrest of the heart, especially if a prolonged ischemic time is anticipated. In this case, the patient's prior coronary operation and the presence of severe aortic insufficiency combined with an inherently complex operation make antegrade delivery of cardioplegia (whether through the pressurized root or through an ostial injection) inadequate [1]. The initial induction dose will fail to pressurize the aortic root given the significant aortic insufficiency. In addition, direct ostial cardioplegia infusion will fail to perfuse the anterolateral wall which, in this case, is supplied extra-anatomically via the LIMA graft. Consequently, retrograde cardioplegia was necessary to achieve adequate myocardial protection [2, 3].

Even the most experienced surgeon will occasionally fail to insert a retrograde cardioplegia cannula into the coronary sinus. This could be because of a small sinus orifice or more often because of an exuberant Chiari network. The use of transesophageal echocardiography (TEE) can help reduce cardiac manipulation and direct atraumatic coronary sinus cannulation in addition to confirming the depth of the cannula tip in relation to the ostium [4]. Additionally, the size of the sinus can be accurately measured via TEE. If a sinus of less than 8 mm or so is present, a smaller catheter with a manually inflated balloon might be squeezed into place whereas a larger catheter with a self-inflating balloon may not fit through the orifice. If all such attempts are futile, snaring the SVC and IVC and opening the right atrium provides direct exposure of the coronary sinus, and a catheter can be secured in place using a purse string. The catheter balloon is then inflated and the catheter is carefully pulled back until the balloon is trapped at the sinus entrance by the purse string [5]. This method provides excellent myocardial protection since it effectively eliminates the "Achilles Heel" of retrograde cardioplegia, namely, the advancement of the catheter tip past some important coronary vein tributaries, resulting in inadequate delivery of cardioplegia to the myocardial territory that these veins drain. What is unacceptable is trying to get by with inadequate protection!

An alternative approach for myocardial protection in patients with prior ITA grafts is systemic cooling leaving the ITA uncontrolled to perfuse the bed of the left anterior descending coronary artery while cardioplegia is delivered retrograde to the remainder of the heart. This has been demonstrated to be effective in the circumstance of aortic valve replacement following prior coronary bypass by several authors [6, 7]. It requires attention to maintaining an adequate systolic pressure for perfusion of the ITA distribution and regular delivery of retrograde cardioplegia to manage the remaining myocardium. The degree of systemic cooling required is a matter of controversy and is not well substantiated by the data, but is commonly to the level of 32 to 34 degrees. In this particular case, given the complexity of the operation anticipated, this is less desirable than controlling the ITA and maintaining complete electromechanical silence.

References

1. Gundry SR, Razzouk AJ, Vigesaa RE, Wang N, Bailey LL. Optimal delivery of cardioplegic solution for "redo" operations. J Thorac Cardiovasc Surg. 1992;103(5):896–901 PMID: 1569772.
2. Mehasche P, Subayi JB, Piwnica A. Retrograde coronary sinus cardioplegia for aortic valve operations: a clinical report on 500 patients. Ann Thoracic Surg. 1990;49:556–64. https://www.annalsthoracicsurgery.org/article/0003-4975(90)90301-L/pdf.
3. Nirupama T, Gerald L, Nan E, De Bakey M. Can retrograde cardioplegia alone provide adequate protection for cardiac valve surgery? CHEST J. 1999;115(1):135–9.
4. Aldea GS, Connelly G, Fonger JD, Dobnick D, Shemin RJ. Directed atraumatic coronary sinus cannulation for retrograde cardioplegia administration. Ann Thorac Surg. 1992;54(4):789–90. https://doi.org/10.1016/0003-4975(92)91036-9 PMID: 1417247.
5. Chitwood WR. Retrograde cardioplegia: current methods. Ann Thorac Surg. 1992;52:352–5.
6. LaPar DJ, Yang Z, Stukenborg GJ, Peeler BB, Kern JA, Kron IL, Ailawadi G. Outcomes of reoperative aortic valve replacement after previous sternotomy. J Thorac Cardiovasc Surg. 2010;139(2):263–72. https://doi.org/10.1016/j.jtcvs.2009.09.006 PMID: 20006357.
7. Park CB, Suri RM, Burkhart HM, Greason KL, Dearani JA, Schaff HV, Sundt TM 3rd. What is the optimal myocardial preservation strategy at re-operation for aortic valve replacement in the presence of a patent internal thoracic artery? Eur J Cardiothorac Surg. 2011;39(6):861–5. https://doi.org/10.1016/j.ejcts.2010.11.007 PMID: 2122771.

Chapter 14
Empty Venous Reservoir

Myles E. Lee and Thoralf M. Sundt

Problem

You have been asked to consult on an obese 83-year-old patient admitted to the ICU in transfer from another hospital with acute shortness of breath. Physical exam on admission was notable for scattered rales. Doppler echocardiography revealed 4 + mitral insufficiency with flail posterior leaflet and a hyperdynamic left ventricle. Cardiac catheterization demonstrated normal coronary arteries. Shortly after her catheterization the patient suddenly became hypotensive, tachycardic and tachypneic requiring expeditious admission to the Cardiac Intensive Care Unit. The cardiology team thinks the contrast load "pushed her over the edge" and now they are pushing you to operate! You consider a temporizing intra-aortic balloon pump, but you catch yourself remembering the last octogenarian vasculopath that showered his feet with cholesterol emboli after a balloon. Instead you recommend an emergency operation. A mechanical problem requires a mechanical solution.

At surgery, her heart rate is 110, the right atrial pressure is 29 mm Hg, and the cardiac index is 1.3 L/min/m^2. The patient sustains another episode of profound hypotension shortly after endotracheal intubation and you ask for full-dose heparin as you prep, drape and rapidly perform a sternotomy. You opt for a 24 French aortic perfusion cannula and a 51-36 double caged venous drainage cannula to quickly get on bypass.

The great vessels are normal, the right atrium somewhat dilated, and the ventricles of normal size and contractility with no evidence of transmural infarction. Almost immediately after you begin cardiopulmonary bypass, however, your per-

M. E. Lee
Department of Cardiothoracic Surgery, Centinela Hospital Medical Center,
Inglewood, CA, USA

T. M. Sundt (✉)
Division of Cardiac Surgery, Massachusetts General Hospital, Boston, MA, USA
e-mail: tsundt@mgh.harvard.edu

© The Author(s), under exclusive license to Springer Nature Switzerland AG 2022   55
T. M. Sundt et al. (eds.), *Near Misses in Cardiac Surgery*,
https://doi.org/10.1007/978-3-030-92750-9_14

fusionists informs you of a rapidly falling blood level in the oxygenator and that he has reached the point where he is no longer able to maintain adequate perfusion. You feel that bone chilling numbness that rises from your feet and courses through your body to the fingertips when you sense that something is terribly wrong and everyone is watching.

Solution

You notice that the right side of the heart has become dramatically dilated and is not being decompressed by the venous cannula. You quickly ascertain that there are no kinks in the venous line, no clamps on the line, and the tip of the venous cannula appears to be in the proper position in the inferior vena cava. As you palpate the vena cava, however, you sense it has a spongy soft feeling that is just not quite right. Still unsure of the underlying cause, you decide that it is time for a change!

You elect to replace the two-stage cannula with separate superior and inferior vena cava cannulas. You place a purse-string suture just above the junction of the superior vena cava with the right atrium, connect two single-stage venous drainage cannulas to a Y connector and interrupt cardiopulmonary bypass. You clamp the two-stage venous cannula and cut it off of the venous line to make room for the Y connector. After clamping the new IVC cannula, you insert the other cannula into the SVC to restore venous return to the oxygenator. Now at least you have partial flow. Next you remove the two-stage cannula, amazed to see it is followed by four separate organized thrombi, each 10 cm long and 1 cm in diameter. They look like casts of the deep femoral or pelvic veins! You quickly insert the new IVC cannula and restore full flow with marked decompression of the right side of the heart. After taking a few deep breaths you proceed with mitral repair.

Discussion

The impaired right-sided decompression in this case resulted from occlusion of a two-stage venous drainage cannula by multiple emboli from the pelvic veins and deep venous system of the lower extremities. It is likely that the patient's episodes of hypotension precipitating both her arrival in the operating room and the necessity for rapid entry into the chest shortly after intubation resulted from recurrent pulmonary emboli. The fact that only mild bibasilar rales could be heard on admission was more consistent with this diagnosis than with an exacerbation of mitral insufficiency which should have been associated with florid pulmonary edema despite the aggressiveness of any prior diuresis. The mitral valve itself revealed only myxomatous degeneration.

Other causes of impaired venous return include malpositioning of the two-stage cannula such that its tip is in the right ventricle instead of the inferior vena cava, or perforation of the inferior vena cava by the tip of the cannula with the cannula itself obstructing flow from the vena cava. It is even possible to impact a relatively small dual stage cannula in a very patulous coronary sinus ostium. With 2 separate venous cannulas, impaired venous return can result from snaring of the superior and/or inferior vena cava with tapes placed beyond the tips of the cannulas, effectively ligating the vena cava. It can also result from failure to drain blood from a left superior vena cava draining into the coronary sinus or placement of a cannula too far into the cavae so as to obstruct venous return from the azygous vein or the hepatic veins. Conversely, an SVC cannula directed posteriorly will impact in the azygous vein. Common to both methods of cannulation, impaired venous drainage may result from kinks in the venous line; a clamp left on the venous line; and an air lock that impedes gravity drainage into the oxygenator with air entry into the line from around an atrial pursestring suture or an unrecognized tear, usually at the junction of the innominate vein with the superior vena cava; or an acute intraoperative aortic dissection.

Bibliography

1. Schabel RK, Berryessa RG, Justison GA, Tyndal CM, Schumann J. Ten common perfusion problems: prevention and treatment protocols. 987. J Extra Corpor Technol. 2007;39:203–9.
2. Matte GS, Howe RJ, Pigula F. A single-center experience with luminal venous cannulae obstruction caused by clot formation during bypass. J Extra Corpor Technol. 2013;45(1):55–7. PMID: 23691786

Chapter 15
Arrest on Induction

Sameer Lakha and Michael G. Fitzsimons

Problem

Having successfully concluded your first case of the day, you greet your second patient before running to your office to catch up on paperwork and dictations. Between the operating room turnover time and induction of anesthesia, you imagine you might even have time to take lunch. Your second case will be a three-vessel coronary bypass in a patient with a preserved ejection fraction. What a great way to end the day! Cardiac catherization showed a right-dominant circulation with 75% occlusion of the left main coronary artery and 90% stenosis of the posterior descending artery. Aside from mildly elevated mean pulmonary artery pressures in the high 20 s, the rest of his cardiac workup was unconcerning.

Your thoughts are brusquely interrupted by your pager. The message is garbled: is the operating room "ready" for you, or do they "need" you? Either way, back to the operating suite you go.

You sense a kerfuffle before even entering the OR. The scene is tense. Your routine second case is in cardiac arrest before the procedure has even started. The operating room team is performing chest compressions. The anesthesiologist tells you that the central line placement was uncomplicated, as was the subsequent induction of anesthesia a few minutes ago. A standard cocktail of narcotic, induction agent, and muscle relaxant, was followed shortly thereafter by pre-operative antibiotic prophylaxis. Just like every other case. No one saw this sudden hemodynamic collapse coming. Before the anesthesiologist can provide more details, the circulating nurse runs over to ask if they should call the hospital "code team." Your heart sinks—a roller-coaster from high to low—what a way to start a case.

S. Lakha · M. G. Fitzsimons (✉)
Division of Cardiac Anesthesia, Department of Anesthesia, Critical Care, and Pain Medicine, Massachusetts General Hospital, Boston, MA, USA
e-mail: mfitzsimons@mgh.harvard.edu

© The Author(s), under exclusive license to Springer Nature Switzerland AG 2022   59
T. M. Sundt et al. (eds.), *Near Misses in Cardiac Surgery*,
https://doi.org/10.1007/978-3-030-92750-9_15

"No need," you reply. Your team is on home turf, and familiar faces at home in the operating room environment are the best ones to manage the patient here. You ask the circulator to grab a colleague from down the hall for an extra set of hands, and the anesthesiologist does the same. In times of crisis it is best to set a number of minds on the problem. The perfusionist is circulating the lines and handing off cannulae while you prep and drape the patient. The chest compressions are effective for now, but muscles fatigue: machines don't.

The anesthesia team is relaying data from their monitors and the echocardiogram. There is no surface ultrasound evidence of pneumothorax from the central line placement; no cardiac tamponade on the echocardiogram; no evidence of acute right ventricular strain. They report adequate ventilation, but keep re-checking the position of the endotracheal tube and commenting on how the lungs feel non-compliant. A widespread rash that appears to be urticaria is noted. Phenylephrine and vasopressin are administered.

Spontaneous circulation has returned as well, but with tenuous hemodynamics in the face of high doses of vasopressor. You are ready to open the chest "crash on pump," still without a clear etiology for this surprising hemodynamic collapse.

"Wait!" In a moment of relative calm, one of the anesthesiologists reviewed the medication record and noted that the cardiac arrest occurred not two minutes after the perioperative antibiotics were administered.

Solution

The medical record indicates that the patient has a history of anaphylaxis to beta-lactam medications. The combination of hypotension, urticaria, wheezing, and bronchospasm points towards anaphylaxis. The patient is placed on 100% oxygen, volume is administered in the form of crystalloid and a bolus of epinephrine (200 mcg) is administered followed by a continuous infusion. Secondary treatment includes antihistamines and corticosteroids. Inhaled beta-2 agonists are given. A serum tryptase level is sent to the lab. Hemodynamic status improves, and the team agrees that a delay for another day is best for the patient and supporting staff.

Discussion

Anaphylaxis is one potential cause of perioperative cardiac arrest. Cardiac surgical patients are exposed to many interventions that place them at risk including antibiotics, blood products, polypeptides such as heparin, and volume-expanding agents.

Anaphylaxis is not the only cause of arrest in the perioperative period. Data on intraoperative cardiac arrest are sparse; fewer data are available specific to the cardiac surgical population. Estimates of incidence among all surgical patients are typically less than 1 in 1,000 cases, although one study identified a rate as high as 0.35% in patients undergoing intrathoracic procedures. Risk factors for perioperative arrest include neonates, children and older age, higher ASA status, trauma, and emergency procedures. Most perioperative arrests are attributed to airway difficulties followed by medications. When intraoperative cardiac arrest does occur, however, it is associated with increased morbidity and mortality.

Cardiac surgical patients that may be particularly at risk include those with pulmonary hypertension and right heart dysfunction, aortic stenosis with reduced ejection fraction, hypertrophic obstructive cardiomyopathy (HOCM) with systolic anterior motion (SAM) of the mitral valve, cardiac tamponade, and significant left main coronary artery disease. Pulmonary hypertension and right heart dysfunction can dramatically worsen in the face of the hypercarbia and vasodilatation that can accompany anesthetic induction due to increased pulmonary vascular resistance and impaired right ventricular perfusion. Patients with "low-flow, low-gradient" aortic stenosis may arrest due to worsening ventricular contractility associated with certain induction agents. A reduction in ventricular preload and peripheral vasodilation may worsen obstruction and SAM in patients with HOCM. Patients in cardiac tamponade or with other obstructive pathology can similarly decompensate rapidly with the drop in ventricular preload seen when anesthesia is induced and positive-pressure ventilation initiated. Significant disease of the left main coronary artery is also particularly susceptible to the hemodynamic changes wrought by the induction of general anesthesia.

In the absence of rigorous research or guidelines, prudence guides the preparatory steps to take in these high-risk patients. All team members should be aware of the heightened risk and understand their role in emergency response. Appropriate invasive monitors and adequate IV access along with medications to offset hemodynamic changes associated with induction are critical. External defibrillator pads can be applied and connected in patients at risk for heart block or that may require external pacing. Bypass equipment should be prepared and personnel stationed in the operating room during anesthetic induction. Femoral arterial and venous access established prior to induction can facilitate emergency bypass or extracorporeal membranous oxygenation (ECMO). Monitoring in cardiac surgical patients facilitates early recognition of deterioration as well as potential causes. Transesophageal echocardiography may reveal previously unsuspected cardiac pathology.

Effective resuscitation begins with high-quality chest compressions and appropriate medical therapy. The cardiac surgical suite allows for rapid institution of extra-corporeal circulation – a step that relieves the task burden on team members, and allows you to address any surgically correctable cardiac pathology that may be the culprit.

Where surgically correctable pathology is not the cause of arrest, and spontaneous circulation is achieved, the question remains whether surgery should proceed as planned once the etiology is identified and treated, or should the patient recover, wake up, and try again later? While correcting surgical pathology could spare the patient the need for another high-risk induction in the future, post-cardiac arrest syndrome arising from whole-body ischemia and reperfusion can lead to multiple organ dysfunction over 48 to 72 h, independent of a run of cardiopulmonary bypass. Awakening the patient instead of proceeding would allow for the evaluation of neurologic status or the potential institution of targeted temperature management if otherwise appropriate. Predictive scores exist to guide prognostication after cardiac arrest, but these have not been specifically validated in the cardiac surgical population. There are no clear answers, and the decision should be made in conjunction with the anesthesiologist, primary cardiologist, and patient's family members.

Bibliography

1. An JX, Zhang LM, Sullivan EA, Guo QL, Williams JP. Interoperative cardiac arrest during anesthesia: a retrospective study of 218,274 anesthetics undergoing non-cardiac surgery in a US teaching hospital. Chinese Med Journal. 2011;124:227–32.
2. Awad H, Smith S, Shehata I, Saklayen S. Con: adult cardiac surgery should not proceed in the event of cardiac arrest after induction of anesthesia. J Card Vasc Anesth. 2020;34:1666–8.
3. Mongardon N, Dumas F, Ricome S, Grimaldi D, Hissem T, Pene F, Cariou A. Postcardiac arrest syndrome: from immediate resuscitation to long-term outcome. Ann Intensive Care. 2011;1–45.
4. Levy JH, Adkinson NF. Anaphylaxis during cardiac surgery: implications for clinicians. Anesth Analg. 2008;106:392–403.
5. Nunnally ME, O'Connor MF, Kordylewski H, Westlake B, Dutton RP. The incidence and risk factors for perioperative cardiac arrest observed in the national anesthesia clinical outcomes registry. Anesth Analg. 2015;120:364–70.
6. Rasul K, Awadallah D, Mathieu W, Bhandary S. Pro: adult cardiac surgery should proceed in the event of cardiac arrest after induction of anesthesia. J Card Vasc Anesth. 2020;34:1663–5.

Chapter 16
Extracorporeal Cardiopulmonary Resuscitation

Jerome C. Crowley

Problem

Availability, affability and ability. You learned that these are the keys to building a practice, so you take every opportunity to review the coronary angiogram of a diabetic patient who has just undergone catheterization for non-ST segment myocardial infarction (NSTEMI) with one of your cardiology colleagues when your concentration is interrupted by an overhead code alarm going off in another room in the catheterization laboratory. Hurrying over to the room, you arrive to see CPR in progress while the code team is securing the patient's airway with an endotracheal tube. One of the nurses fills you in on the background; a male patient in his 50s presented with crushing chest pain and ST elevations in the anterior leads. While attempting to engage the left coronary artery, the patient went into ventricular tachycardia which quickly degenerated into ventricular fibrillation. Pulsatility is only noted on the arterial line during chest compressions and the ventricular fibrillation persists despite anti-arrhythmics and defibrillation per advanced cardiac life support (ACLS) protocols.

Recognizing a potentially salvageable situation, you immediately activate the ECMO team and scrub in to help with cannulation. After obtaining arterial and venous access, you place appropriately sized cannulae under fluoroscopic guidance and connect them to the ECMO circuit. With extracorporeal support initiated, an immediate improvement in hemodynamics is noted with a decline in the Levophed dose and conversion to a slow junctional rhythm. The patient's mottled appearance is already beginning to improve. You begin to break scrub so the interventionalists can get back to work assessing the patient's coronary artery disease when the respiratory therapist starts to express concern over the volume of pulmonary edema emanating from the endotracheal tube. You walk to the head of the table to assess

J. C. Crowley (✉)
Department of Anesthesia, Massachusetts General Hospital, Boston, MA, USA
e-mail: jccrowley@mgh.harvard.edu

© The Author(s), under exclusive license to Springer Nature Switzerland AG 2022
T. M. Sundt et al. (eds.), *Near Misses in Cardiac Surgery*,
https://doi.org/10.1007/978-3-030-92750-9_16

the situation with the intensivist and witness a non-stop torrent of pink-tinged frothy fluid that shows no signs of abating despite positive end-expiratory pressure. Fluoroscopy of the chest reveals an appropriately positioned endotracheal tube but significant pulmonary edema. In addition, despite restoration of normal mean arterial blood pressure, the patient persists in ventricular fibrillation. To make matters worse, the ECMO circuit is starting to chatter and the intensivists request more volume, but the severe pulmonary edema makes you hesitate. Post-cannulation arterial blood gas reveals an arterial saturation of 79%. You can see the resident scratching her head—isn't ECMO supposed to fix this problem?

Pulmonary artery catheterization reveals low central venous pressure (CVP) but elevated pulmonary artery diastolic pressure. STAT echocardiography is ordered to rule out effusion and none is noted. At this time, the respiratory therapist has resorted to clamping the endotracheal tube to stop the ongoing volume loss. You realize you must act quickly to salvage viable myocardium to give the patient a chance to recover.

Solution

Echocardiography reveals the problem immediately; the left ventricle is severely distended with significant mitral regurgitation noted and no organized contractility. After a quick discussion with your interventional cardiology colleague, you both decide the appropriate course of action is to place a left ventricular vent to decompress the left ventricle. Arterial access is obtained in the contralateral common femoral artery and a percutaneous ventricular assist device is placed in the left ventricle across the aortic valve with its position confirmed by fluoroscopy and echocardiography.

Ventricular assist device support is initiated at a low level and almost immediately the pulmonary artery diastolic pressure begins to decrease. Another attempt is made at defibrillation and this time the patient converts to sinus rhythm with a left bundle branch block. Cautious unclamping of the endotracheal tube reveals significant resolution of the edema and lung protective ventilation is successfully initiated.

Now satisfied that the patient is stable from a cardiopulmonary standpoint, you turn over the rest of the care to your interventional colleagues who immediately get to work opening a likely culprit lesion in the left anterior descending artery. As you leave the catherization laboratory, one of the nurses waves goodbye and says "it would be great to always have a cardiac surgeon up here."

Discussion

Veno-arterial extracorporeal membrane oxygenation during cardiopulmonary resuscitation, termed E-CPR, has significant potential to allow for good recovery from otherwise fatal events. Of particular interest is refractory VT/VF arrest from coronary artery disease as this disease process responds well to CPR and has a rapidly reversible solution if prompt cardiac catheterization can be performed. Several factors play into the likelihood of recovery, the most important of which is minimization of downtime without CPR (referred to as "no-flow time"). However, it is critical to recognize that while VA ECMO will stabilize the patient and hopefully prevent end organ injury, it does not treat the underlying coronary artery disease and in a poorly contractile heart the increase in afterload from the retrograde flow from the ECMO circuit will result in *increased* myocardial oxygen consumption. This in turn will lead to left ventricular distension and consequently severe pulmonary edema. If this is not reversed, injury to the heart and lungs becomes permanent.

The solution to this problem is twofold; first, venting the left ventricle to reduce distension and second, coronary angiography to identify and potentially restore perfusion to acutely ischemic myocardium. Left ventricular venting can be accomplished by a variety of techniques. The first involves placing a surgical vent in the pulmonary veins; however, this requires a surgical incision and is not well suited to an emergent procedure in a patient who is most likely not in the operating room. A second method is to perform a septostomy to decompress the left side; until recently this was the standard method of left ventricular decompression in the emergent setting. A newer technique is to place a percutaneous left ventricular assist device to decompress the left ventricle. This method has the benefit of not leaving an atrial septal defect and may help with weaning from ECMO as the right heart and pulmonary function recover. The drawback is the expertise required to place the device, the expense, and the chance of complications from the device. As a normal size heart recovers from stunning, it may begin to contract and contact the percutaneous VAD triggering significant ectopy and arrythmias. The treatment for these arrhythmias is removal of the device if adequate position cannot be achieved.

Similar to the operating room post cardiopulmonary bypass, a distended heart is unlikely to convert to sinus rhythm owing to increased left ventricular wall tension. Prompt decompression is critical to reduce myocardial oxygen consumption and resultant infarct burden on the heart.

Bibliography

1. Sidebotham D. Troubleshooting adult ECMO. J Extra Corpor Technol. 2011;43(1):P27-32 PMID: 21449237.
2. Vallabhajosyula S, O'Horo JC, Antharam P, Ananthaneni S, Vallabhajosyula S, Stulak JM, Dunlay SM, Holmes DR Jr, Barsness GW. Venoarterial extracorporeal membrane oxygenation with concomitant impella versus venoarterial extracorporeal membrane oxygenation for cardiogenic shock. ASAIO J. 2020;66(5):497–503. https://doi.org/10.1097/MAT.0000000000001039 PMID: 31335363.
3. Grajeda Silvestri ER, Pino JE, Donath E, Torres P, Chait R, Ghumman W. Impella to unload the left ventricle in patients undergoing venoarterial extracorporeal membrane oxygenation for cardiogenic shock: a systematic review and meta-analysis. J Card Surg. 2020;35(6):1237–42.
4. Yannopoulos D, Bartos J, Raveendran G, Walser E, Connett J, Murray TA, Collins G, Zhang L, Kalra R, Kosmopoulos M, John R, Shaffer A, Frascone RJ, Wesley K, Conterato M, Biros M, Tolar J, Aufderheide TP. Advanced reperfusion strategies for patients with out-of-hospital cardiac arrest and refractory ventricular fibrillation (ARREST): a phase 2, single centre, open-label, randomised controlled trial. Lancet. 2020;396(10265):1807–16.

Chapter 17
Postoperative Hypotension in the ICU

Myles E. Lee and Thoralf M. Sundt

Problem

You have performed uneventful coronary artery bypass grafting on a 73-year-old patient with triple-vessel coronary disease and normal left ventricular function. During the first 6 postoperative hours, a liter of blood drains from the chest tubes. Despite vigorous volume replacement, the blood pressure remains 85 mmHg systolic, with right atrial, pulmonary artery, and pulmonary capillary wedge pressures of 10, 20/13, and 13 mm Hg, respectively. You start a dopamine drip, but the cardiac index rises no higher than 1.83 L/min/m^2, and the patient becomes oliguric. The electrocardiogram is normal, but a repeat chest roentgenogram demonstrates some mediastinal widening with obscuration of the right pulmonary artery, which, previously, had been clearly seen. Physical examination reveals distention of the cervical veins despite the low filling pressures. A quick bedside surface ECHO using the mini-ultrasound machine the intensivists have just introduced shows no pericardial effusion around the LV! Right before your eyes, almost defiantly, this patient, with normal biventricular function, is choosing the path of least resistance straight down a black hole from which nothing, not even light, is known to escape, and you are about to follow him unless you can think of something fast.

M. E. Lee
Department of Cardiac Surgery, Centinela Hospital Medical Center, Inglewood, CA, USA

T. M. Sundt (✉)
Division of Cardiac Surgery, Massachusetts General Hospital, Boston, MA, USA
e-mail: tsundt@mgh.harvard.edu

© The Author(s), under exclusive license to Springer Nature Switzerland AG 2022   67
T. M. Sundt et al. (eds.), *Near Misses in Cardiac Surgery*,
https://doi.org/10.1007/978-3-030-92750-9_17

Solution

Suspicious of pericardial tamponade, although the hemodynamics did not display the usual elevation and equalization of pressures, you return the patient to the operating room where you find a 6 cm clot has compressed the junction of the superior vena cava and right atrium like a Brobdingnagian fist. Upon removing the clot, the arterial pressure shoots up to 190 mmHg, requiring control with nitroprusside. A postoperative chest roentgenogram reveals a narrower cardiac silhouette with restored visibility of the right pulmonary artery. The remainder of the patient's course is entirely uneventful.

Discussion

Pericardial tamponade from nonsurgical effusions (uremic, malignant) tends to produce relatively uniform compression of all cardiac chambers with a circumferential distribution. The classically described elevation and equalization of pressures in pericardial tamponade requires equal compression of all chambers by a uniformly distributed volume of liquid within the relatively inelastic pericardium. During inspiration the increased venous return filling the right ventricle limits left ventricular filling, reduces cardiac output, and causes subendocardial ischemia. During expiration the wedge pressure increases, temporarily enhancing left ventricular filling and cardiac output. This mechanism accounts for the *pulsus paradoxus* seen with pericardial tamponade.

After cardiac surgery, however, asymmetric compression of a single cardiac chamber may impair cardiac output without the expected hemodynamic pattern. This patient demonstrated an acute superior vena cava syndrome caused by a huge clot that compressed the superior vena cava and restricted flow into the right atrium. Thus, the cervical venous pressure was elevated, and the right atrial and pulmonary artery pressures remained within normal limits despite aggressive volume replacement.

Asymmetric, nonuniform single chamber tamponade is the rule, rather than the exception, following cardiac surgery. The final common pathway of all tamponade is hypotension and depressed cardiac output, but the hemodynamic patterns can have discrete characteristics. For example, right atrial tamponade is characterized by elevated right atrial pressure in the presence of normal pulmonary artery and pulmonary capillary pressures. It may be necessary to challenge the patient with volume to magnify this difference. Case reports of compression of the pulmonary outflow tract, left atrium, and left ventricle have also been well described.

In years past, Technetium 99-m ventriculography was useful for differentiating biventricular failure from pericardial tamponade but is not applicable in a setting such as described here. Transesophageal echocardiography has become the gold standard and can give an excellent view of a localized thrombus causing focal compression including right atrial compression or left atrial compression, which can be even more subtle, but one has to look for it. Although hand-held echocardiographic devices are increasingly used, they do not provide as good image resolution as a transthoracic probe.

The treatment of postoperative pericardial tamponade requires prompt diagnosis and intervention as a lifesaving maneuver. Early in the postoperative period pericardial tamponade must be anticipated in the patient with unexpected unexplained hemodynamic instability and normal ventricular function. Importantly, if not caught sufficiently early, a long slow slide of hypotension can lead to pulseless electrical activity (PEA) or ventricular fibrillation, the treatment of which is to open the chest immediately. External compressions will be ineffective in the setting of tamponade, so no time should be wasted before opening the chest. One is wise to remember the advice of a senior surgeon "Sinus rhythm … no blood pressure … open the chest." Conversely, however, if tamponade is not a leading diagnosis, it is worthwhile being somewhat circumspect before reopening the chest in settings where arrhythmia may be the cause, perhaps, and only an external shock would be effective.

Late tamponade usually occurs in patients on anticoagulants and should be suspected in patients who may appear septic or simply "not doing well." Late effusions can often be dealt with percutaneously under fluoroscopic or echocardiographic guidance.

Bibliography

1. Lee MD, Gray RJ. Low output state following cardiac surgery. In: Gray RJ, Matloff JM, editors. Medical Management of the Cardiac Surgical Patient. Baltimore: Williams and Wilkins; 1990. p. 147–51.
2. Hutchins GM, Moore GW. Isolated right atrial tamponade caused by hematoma complicating coronary artery bypass graft surgery. Arch Path Lab Med. 1980;104:612–4.
3. Yacoub MH, Cleveland WP, Deal CW. Left atrial tamponade. Thorax. 1966;21:305–9.
4. Ashikhmina EA, Schaff HV, Sinak LJ, Li Z, Dearani JA, Suri RM, Park SJ, Orszulak TA, Sundt TM 3rd. Pericardial effusion after cardiac surgery: risk factors, patient profiles, and contemporary management. Ann Thorac Surg. 2010;89(1):112–8. https://doi.org/10.1016/j.athoracsur.2009.09.026.
5. The society of thoracic surgeons expert consensus for the resuscitation of patients who arrest after cardiac surgery. Ann Thorac Surg. 2017;103(3):1005–20. https://doi.org/10.1016/j.athoracsur.2016.10.033. Epub 2017 Jan 22.

Chapter 18
Hemodynamic Instability After Pulmonary Thromboendarterectomy

Asishana Osho and Nathaniel B. Langer

Problem

Your first patient in the operating room this week is a 38-year-old woman with ulcerative colitis (UC) whose last abdominal operation was complicated by a significant pulmonary embolus approximately two months postoperatively. She recovered following thrombolysis but was referred to your office in the setting of progressive dyspnea, elevated pulmonary artery pressures, and imaging evidence of significant chronic thromboembolic pulmonary hypertension (CTEPH). After a complete pre-operative workup, including confirmation of her UC maintenance medication regime, you schedule her for a pulmonary thromboendarterectomy. You perform the operation successfully with periods of intermittent circulatory arrest, producing a completely intact network of pulmonary thrombus on both sides. You take photos and send them to your mentor from fellowship. He will most certainly be proud of this one!

Three hours later you start to wonder whether you should have been so quick to pat yourself on the back. After separating from bypass without issue and a smooth transition to the ICU, your patient developed hypotension that thus far has been refractory to catecholamines and robust fluid resuscitation. Workup ruled out hemorrhage, and her hemodynamics are not suggestive of tamponade. In fact, she appears profoundly vasodilated. Suspecting sepsis, you start broad spectrum antibiotics but are left wondering what else could be contributing to this presentation.

A. Osho · N. B. Langer (✉)
Department of Surgery, Massachusetts General Hospital, Boston, MA, USA
e-mail: Nlanger@partners.org

A. Osho
e-mail: Asishana.osho@mgh.harvard.edu

© The Author(s), under exclusive license to Springer Nature Switzerland AG 2022
T. M. Sundt et al. (eds.), *Near Misses in Cardiac Surgery*,
https://doi.org/10.1007/978-3-030-92750-9_18

Solution

Fortunately, you were diligent in your preoperative evaluation and aware that her UC treatment included maintenance dose steroids. Even though the dose was low, you brought it up during the preoperative huddle and the patient received intravenous stress dose steroids after induction. Despite this, you begin to suspect your patient is suffering from relative adrenal insufficiency following cardiopulmonary bypass. At your request, an additional dose of hydrocortisone is administered, and a cortisol level is sent. To your delight, it's not long before the patient's hemodynamics improve. She is weaned off catecholamines by the next morning and transferred out of the ICU by POD3. She is discharged home a week and a half after the operation on a slow steroid taper.

Discussion

The hypothalamus–pituitary–adrenal axis is a critical actor in the maintenance of homeostasis following surgery. Postoperative adrenal insufficiency manifests as immediate or delayed postoperative hemodynamic instability refractory to vasoactive medications and fluid resuscitation. Patients can present with a wide range of clinical and laboratory abnormalities including altered mental status, lethargy, nausea, fever, tachycardia, bradycardia, hyponatremia, and hyperkalemia. Patients at risk for postoperative adrenal insufficiency include those with primary (adrenal gland pathology), secondary (pituitary-hypothalamic pathology), or tertiary adrenal insufficiency (relative global suppression due to long-term exogenous steroid therapy). Given the vast array of chronic conditions that are managed with steroids, tertiary adrenal insufficiency is the most common etiology encountered postoperatively.

Recognizing patients at risk for adrenal insufficiency is critical in minimizing the risk of adrenal crises. A patient on chronic steroids (greater than one month) with daily doses greater than the equivalent of 5 mg of prednisone should be considered to have relative suppression of the hypothalamic–pituitary–adrenal axis. Measures to prevent adrenal crises in these patients should include increasing the baseline dose a few days prior to surgery, administering intravenous high-dose steroids during induction, and initiating a maintenance regimen of intravenous steroids intraoperatively and postoperatively until the patient can be steadily tapered back to their maintenance dose.

When adrenal crises do occur, the management is steroid replacement as expediently as possible. 100 mg IV hydrocortisone administered every 6 to 12 h is typically adequate coverage (4 mg IV dexamethasone is a reasonable alternative but has no mineralocorticoid activity and may be inadequate for patients with primary adrenal insufficiency). As the presentation of adrenal insufficiency is somewhat non-specific, with features that could mimic more common postoperative issues, a high index of suspicion is critical in patients with increased risk. During cardiopulmonary bypass, the pump can be used to control associated electrolyte and volume changes, but it is also reasonable to re-dose intravenous steroids in the right clinical context. Serum evaluation with free cortisol and ACTH stimulation testing could be helpful, but administration of steroids should not be delayed for laboratory testing. Once patients have recovered from the acute episode of insufficiency, a plan can be put in place to taper back to the maintenance dose within 2–7 days depending on the operation and severity of the episode.

Bibliography

1. Serrano N, Jiménez JJ, Brouard MT, Málaga J, Mora ML. Acute adrenal insufficiency after cardiac surgery. Crit Care Med. 2000;28(2):569–70. https://doi.org/10.1097/00003246-200002000-00048.
2. Graham EM, Bradley SM. First nights, the adrenal axis, and steroids. J Thorac Cardiovasc Surg. 2017;153(5):1164–6. https://doi.org/10.1016/j.jtcvs.2016.12.013.
3. Woodcock T, Barker P, Daniel S, et al. Guidelines for the management of glucocorticoids during the peri-operative period for patients with adrenal insufficiency. Anaesthesia. 2020;75 (5):654–63. https://doi.org/10.1111/anae.14963.
4. D'Silva C, Watson D, Ngaage D. A strategy for management of intraoperative Addisonian crisis during coronary artery bypass grafting. Interact Cardiovasc Thorac Surg. 2012;14 (4):481–2. https://doi.org/10.1093/icvts/ivr139.

Chapter 19
Inadequate Venous Drainage

Antonia Kreso and Serguei I. Melnitchouk

Problem

A 57-year-old man known hypertension, hyperlipidemia, type 2 diabetes, and
Gilbert syndrome presented to the emergency ward with chest pain. Unsurprisingly,
given his risk factors, workup revealed multivessel coronary artery disease. There
was chronic total occlusion of the LAD, severe ostial D1, ostial OM2, and distal
RCA disease extending to the ostium of the right PDA. Transthoracic echocardiogram revealed normal left ventricular end diastolic volume, no wall motion
abnormalities, an ejection fraction of 62%, and a patent foramen ovale (PFO).
Despite enthusiasm from your interventional colleagues who have just launched a
"CTO" program for treating chronic total occlusions, the clinical cardiology team
asked for a surgical opinion given the patient's diabetes and young age. You have
been advocating for the long-term value of arterial revascularization of just such
patients, and perhaps you are making some progress! Surgical consultation was
requested, and revascularization with PFO closure was recommended. The patient
agreed.

In the operating room, you take down the LIMA while the left radial artery is
being harvested, planning a composite graft to reach all targets via a "T-Graft"
configuration. After sewing the radial artery to the LITA, you cannulate the aorta
centrally and insert bicaval cannulae. Cardiopulmonary bypass is initiated without
issues. You cross clamp the aorta and give antegrade cardioplegia, achieving a
quick diastolic arrest.

You decide to begin by closing the PFO recognizing that it is easy to forget what
seems an obvious step at the end of a tedious operation. It would be embarrassing to

A. Kreso · S. I. Melnitchouk (✉)
Department of Surgery, Massachusetts General Hospital, Boston, MA, USA
e-mail: Smelnitchouk@mgh.harvard.edu

A. Kreso
e-mail: akreso@mgh.harvard.edu

© The Author(s), under exclusive license to Springer Nature Switzerland AG 2022
T. M. Sundt et al. (eds.), *Near Misses in Cardiac Surgery*,
https://doi.org/10.1007/978-3-030-92750-9_19

have to re-arrest the heart or worsen explain why you did not address this structural abnormality. Tightening the caval snares, it takes only a small incision in the right atrium and a figure-of-eight stitch to address the PFO. After closing the right atrium you position the heart to expose the PDA. Here, you fashion an end-to-side anastomosis of the radial artery to the target vessel in a perpendicular fashion. Next, you rotate the heart to visualize the OM2 target. Focused on getting the inter-graft lengths correct and avoiding any twisting of the radial artery conduit, you open the target vessel before incising the radial only to be disturbed by a complaint from the perfusionist that the venous reservoir is almost empty and they are unable to provide adequate flow. What an awkward moment! And just as you have the heart positioned exactly where you want to do your anastomosis. You ask the perfusionist to recheck the venous lines to make sure there is no kink or obstruction, of which there is none. Reluctantly you release the retractor you had placed to hold the heart in place, but there is still no improvement in venous drainage. The room has come to a quiet stop. But you are anything but quiet inside. You need to come up with a solution. Now!

Solution

You palpate the IVC and confirm that the cannula is still in the correct position. You remove the snare with little improvement but see a dramatic collapse of the right atrium when you pull back the cannula just a few centimeters. Venous drainage immediately improves. You then proceed with the remainder of the operation without issues. You suspect the IVC cannula must have lodged in the hepatic vein on positioning of the heart for bypass. The patient has an uneventful post-operative recovery.

Discussion

There are myriad reasons for poor venous drainage on bypass. Having a systematic method to troubleshoot possible causes is critical. Reasons for poor venous drainage include a venous cannula that is too small, a kink in the line, or a malpositioned cannula. For example, the cannula may be in the right ventricle or coronary sinus. One example is when the venous cannula lodges itself into a hepatic vein. This could potentially lead to disastrous intra-abdominal compartment syndrome if caval tapes are used and this is not recognized early. Likewise, if the femoral vessels are used for cannulation, one must rule out a retroperitoneal bleed. Another example is when a dual stage cannula is used and the heart is elevated for exposure (e.g., for circumflex artery bypass). A simple solution in this situation would be to let down the pericardial sutures on the right side to improve venous drainage.

Another reason for poor venous drainage is a massive airlock within the system. If the amount of air is moderate or small, it can be chased back by progressively lifting the venous line. Alternatively, more vacuum can be applied to the system. If this fails, the cardiopulmonary bypass pump can be stopped, the venous cannula separated from the venous line, and the venous line manually filled with saline. After subsequent reconnection to the venous cannula, cardiopulmonary bypass can be reinitiated. If despite these adjustments, the target flow rate cannot be achieved, one can cool the patient to moderate hypothermia, which decreases metabolic demand, enabling the patient to tolerate a slightly lower flow rate. Often, increasing suction on the venous cannula (or elevating the level of the patient in relation to the reservoir if relying on gravity) can help increase venous drainage.

Bibliography

1. Kirkeby-Garstad I, Tromsdal A, Sellevold OFM, Bjorngaard M, Bjella LK, Berg EM, Karevold A, Haaverstad R, Wahba A, Tjomsland O, Astudillo R, Krogstad A, Stenseth R. Guiding surgical cannulation of the inferior vena cava with trans-esophageal echocardiography. Anesth Analg. 2003;96:1288–93.
2. Mokadam NA. Cardiopulmonary bypass: a primer. University of Washington Division of Cardiothoracic Surgery. Copyright 2015, Apple iBook Store.

Chapter 20
Trapped Mitral Leaflet

Antonia Kreso and Serguei I. Melnitchouk

Problem

A 59-year-old female with history of mitral stenosis and atrial fibrillation presented with progressively worsening shortness of breath and dyspnea on exertion. Transthoracic echocardiography has demonstrated severe mitral stenosis and what looks like rheumatic disease. The referring physician sends cases routinely for mitral repair as she knows your repair rate exceeds 95%; she also appreciates your judicious use of minimally invasive approaches when appropriate. In this case, although she thinks replacement will be necessary, she sends this patient your way. After a visit in your office, you agree with a touch of melancholy. Yes, replacement means you will not experience those anxious moments after the clamp is removed awaiting return of contractility and the evaluation of your success by the echocardiographer on weaning from bypass. But neither will you feel that rush of pleasure when they declare your repairs pure artistry. And on top of it, you have actually become more comfortable with repairs than replacements as time has passed. So, you recommended mitral valve replacement along with left atrial appendage amputation and a Maze procedure. After discussing the risks and benefits of a tissue versus mechanical valve, the patient chose a mechanical prosthesis.

You cannulate the aorta and perform bicaval cannulation. You cross clamp the aorta, administer cardioplegia, and amputate the left atrial appendage. After finishing the left-sided Maze lesions, you examine the valve and find a severely stenotic mitral valve with pronounced thickening of the entire subvalvular apparatus as well as some mild calcification along the posterior annulus. You resect the entire anterior leaflet along with its very thickened chords but preserve most of the

A. Kreso · S. I. Melnitchouk (✉)
Department of Surgery, Massachusetts General Hospital, Boston, MA, USA
e-mail: smelnitchouk@mgh.harvard.edu

A. Kreso
e-mail: akreso@mgh.harvard.edu

© The Author(s), under exclusive license to Springer Nature Switzerland AG 2022
T. M. Sundt et al. (eds.), *Near Misses in Cardiac Surgery*,
https://doi.org/10.1007/978-3-030-92750-9_20

posterior leaflet along with chordal support in preparation for mitral valve replacement. You implant a 29 mm St. Jude bileaflet mechanical prosthesis. Happy with the result, you close the left atrium, de-air, and wean from bypass. Upon examining the valve using trans-esophageal echocardiography, the anesthesia team reports, much to your dismay, that one of the leaflets is not moving. Everyone in the room becomes as motionless as the valve leaflet and looks at you for an answer. You gently shake the patient's heart in the desperate hope that both leaflets will start moving; however, the stubbornly stuck leaflet shows no sign of cooperating.

Solution

With a sigh, you go back on full bypass and arrest the heart. You open the left atrium and inspect the valve in a systematic fashion. You open the valve using the back of a Q-tip and look for trapped chords, suture, or some excess tissue. To your dismay, however, you find none of these potential causes. After taking another close look while irrigating the left ventricle with saline, you still cannot find any offending agent. Somewhat puzzled not to find a culprit to blame, you once again examine the valve, and now the leaflets are opening and closing without any apparent issue. You ask the nurse if he still has the valve holder. Your heart starts to sink when he says, "what valve holder?" Luckily, he finds it sterile in the pouch off the Mayo stand. You use the valve holder to rotate the entire valve 45 degrees (does not matter to which side) and test it again, confirming that it continues to be functional and that there is no interaction between leaflet motion and subvalvular structures. You close the left atriotomy once again, wean the patient off bypass, and turn your head to the left. The echocardiographer informs you that the valve is now opening and closing without any issues. You complete the remainder of the case, and the patient has an unremarkable post-operative course.

Discussion

During mitral valve replacement, seating of the valve is dependent on the type of valve used. Mechanical valves should ideally be implanted in an anti-anatomic position, with the hinge lines orthogonal to the mitral valve commissures. This position is preferred to the anatomic placement to avoid the so-called "lazy leaflet" phenomenon. Vector flow mapping studies of left atrial hydraulics have found that when both leaflets of a prosthetic valve are positioned in an anti-anatomic orientation, they receive equal initial opening force owing to the symmetric orientation of the leaflets relative to the atrial vortex [3]. If the valve is placed in anatomic position, the posterior leaflet demonstrates delayed opening and early closure. Studies have also shown that asynchronous leaflet closure is reduced in valves that are implanted in the anti-anatomic position and that anti-anatomic positioning can improve leaflet clearance to the posterior ventricle and decrease the risk of impingement [4]. Similarly, bioprosthetic valves must be carefully oriented with the posts out of the outflow tract facing the trigones and the third post bisecting the posterior leaflet. For both valves, there should be no interference from the sub-valvular apparatus.

A trapped leaflet after a valve replacement can be due to several reasons. Obstruction causing a stuck mechanical valve can be intrinsic or extrinsic. Intrinsic dysfunction can be due to manufacturing defects, which are vanishingly rare, while extrinsic obstruction can be attributed to mitral subvalvular apparatus or suboptimal placement. Other things to consider are trapped chords or suture material. Irrespective of cause, the surgeon needs to meticulously examine the valve in a systematic fashion, looking for these potential offenders. If a problem is not found, rotating the valve 45 degrees is often sufficient to correct a trapped leaflet. If both aortic and mitral valves were replaced and the mitral valve now needs to be examined or possibly replaced, one may need to do this via a transseptal approach to ensure reasonable mitral exposure in the setting of existent aortic valve prosthesis [1, 2].

References

1. Almeida J, Santos A, Barreiros F, Garcia M, Pinho P. Stuck leaflet of bileaflet prosthesis in mitral position – five cases to make us think. Interact Cardiovasc Thorac Surg. 2007;6(3):379–83.
2. Raut MS, Maheshwari A, Dubey S. Intraoperative detection of stuck leaflet of prosthetic mitral valve. Indian Heart J. 2017;69(4):519–22.
3. Deng Y, Belfar A, Powell T. Early prosthetic valve malfunction leading to cardiogenic shock and emergency redo mitral valve replacement. J Cardiothorac Vasc Anesth. 2019;33(10):2866–69.
4. Laub GW, Muralidharan S, Pollock SB, Adkins MS, McGrath LB. The experimental relationship between leaflet clearance and orientation of the St. Jude medical valve in the mitral position. J Thorac Cardiovasc Surg. 1992;103(4): 638–41.

Chapter 21
Even More Complications of TAVR

Asishana Osho and Nathaniel Langer

Problem

Just as you are finishing morning rounds you receive a page from your team notifying you they are ready for you to start your case, a transcatheter aortic valve replacement (TAVR). The last patient you saw on rounds that morning received a TAVR the previous day and was left with a small paravalvular leak (PVL). During the briefing, your fellow outlines the plan for a 75-year-old man with severe aortic stenosis and significant calcification around the annulus. The annular dimensions fall within the acceptable range for two sizes of balloon expandable valves. After some discussion, the team selects the larger valve—no PVL today. You are quite disappointed when the echocardiographer shows you an area of trace mild PVL after deployment. Determined to improve upon yesterday's result, you post-dilate the valve, adding 2 cc to the balloon. On subsequent evaluation of the valve on echocardiography, there is no longer a paravalvular leak. There is, however, a rapidly enlarging hematoma in the aortic root. Subsequent root angiography confirms a contained rupture of the aortic annulus.

Solution

Maintaining your wire position within the ventricle, you quickly withdraw the existing valve deployment system. You have read about percutaneous salvage options, and there is discussion of deploying a second valve to seal the rupture site.

A. Osho · N. Langer (✉)
Department of Surgery, Massachusetts General Hospital, Boston, MA, USA
e-mail: nlanger@mgh.harvard.edu

A. Osho
e-mail: Asishana.osho@mgh.harvard.edu

© The Author(s), under exclusive license to Springer Nature Switzerland AG 2022
T. M. Sundt et al. (eds.), *Near Misses in Cardiac Surgery*,
https://doi.org/10.1007/978-3-030-92750-9_21

Initially, you place a pericardial drain and relieve the tamponade; however, as discussion continues, you notice a progressively enlarging pericardial effusion with ongoing drainage of blood. As continuous transfusion of blood products is required to maintain reasonable perfusion pressures, you decide that an open surgical repair is required. You call your chief resident, who cannulates the femoral vessels for cardiopulmonary bypass while you open the chest. Once the pericardium is open, you immediately note a large root hematoma. After arresting the heart and opening the aorta, you inspect the root for any accompanying coronary injury. Then you remove both TAVR prostheses and perform a patch repair of the annulus with bovine pericardium. You subsequently perform a surgical aortic valve replacement. Thankfully, there are no difficulties separating from bypass, and the patient is extubated that evening. On your drive home, songs from Taylor Swift's latest album prompt you to call your faculty mentor who talks through the case with you and provides much needed reassurance after a difficult day.

Discussion

Aortic or left ventricular outflow tract (LVOT) rupture during TAVR is an uncommon complication, occurring in 0.5–1% of cases. While rare, the associated early mortality is between 25 and 60%. The risk of rupture is highest with balloon expandable valves and during post-deployment dilation of self-expanded prostheses, especially when the prosthesis is over-sized (>20% larger than the annular area) or when there is severe subannular or LVOT calcium. In severe ruptures, the problem is immediately evident owing to hemodynamic decline at the time of valve deployment. Echocardiography is typically the critical diagnostic modality.

The clinical manifestations of TAVR-associated rupture vary with the location and severity of injury. Rupture in the subannular location can create a ventricular septal defect (VSD), mitral valve injury with associated mitral regurgitation, or a left ventricle to right atrium fistula (iatrogenic Gerbode defect). Depending on the degree of injury, these may be managed expectantly, with interventional occluders (for ventricular defects) or with surgical closure. Rupture in the intra-annular location can result in aortic root injury, potentially with coronary involvement requiring open repair and aortic root replacement. Rupture in the supra-annular location can cause intramural hematoma or frank ascending aortic rupture with hemodynamic compromise. Presentations can range from asymptomatic (discovered on routine echocardiography) to immediate hemodynamic instability due to tamponade. For contained ruptures, percutaneous pericardial drainage may provide adequate relief. Open repair is required for free ruptures.

In all cases, interval surveillance imaging is required as even asymptomatic patients may eventually develop progression of the injury. Because of this risk for progression, all therapeutic anticoagulants should be discontinued if possible. There are several reports of managing rupture with deployment of a second valve at the site of the rupture, if it is near the skirt of the existing valve. This approach is only feasible if injury is limited to the annulus without extension into the LVOT and if a second valve can safely be deployed without obstructing the coronary ostia.

Bibliography

1. Langer NB, Hamid NB, Nazif TM, Khalique, Vahl TP, White J, Terre J, Hastings R, Leung, D, Hahn RT, Leon M, Kodali S, George I. Injuries to the aorta, aortic annulus, and left ventricle during transcatheter aortic valve replacement: management and outcomes. Circ Cardiovasc Interv. 2017;10(1):e004735.
2. Coughlan JJ, Kiernan T, Mylotte D, Arnous. Annular rupture during transcatheter aortic valve implantation: predictors, management and outcomes. Interv Cardiol. 2018;13(3):140–4. https://doi.org/10.15420/icr.2018.20.2.
3. Rezq A, Basavarajaiah, Latib A, Takagi K, Hasegawa T, Figini F, Cioni M, Franco A, Montorfano M, Chieffo A, Maisano F, Corvaja N, Alfieri O, Colombo A. Incidence, management, and outcomes of cardiac tamponade during transcatheter aortic valve implantation: a single-center study. JACC Cardiovasc Interv. 2012;5(12):1264–72. https://doi.org/10.1016/j.jcin.2012.08.012.
4. Arsalan M, Kim W-K, Van Linden A, Liebetrau C, Pollock BD, Filardo G, Renker M, Mollmann H, Doss M, Fischer-Rasokat U, Skwara A, Hamm CW, Walther T. Predictors and outcome of conversion to cardiac surgery during transcatheter aortic valve implantation. Eur J Cardiothorac Surg. 2018;54(2):267–72. https://doi.org/10.1093/ejcts/ezy034.

Chapter 22
Conduit for Redo CABG

Brittany Potz and George Tolis

Problem

You're in the middle of clinic when you receive an in-house consult request to evaluate a 56-year-old man for coronary artery disease. Between outpatient visits you reflect on how terrible it is to need coronary bypass at such a young age, but as an all-arterial enthusiast, you are certain you are just the surgeon to take care of him! Then you discover the rest of the story. He underwent a minimally invasive direct coronary bypass for angina four years ago but had recurrence of his symptoms earlier this year. Cardiac catheterization performed via the right radial artery demonstrates a 90% proximal LAD lesion at the site of takeoff of a large first diagonal branch. His circumflex and right coronary arteries show only non-obstructive luminal irregularities. To the cardiologist's surprise, the LITA is anastomosed to the large diagonal instead of the LAD and that anastomosis is widely patent. His BMI is 35, he is a poorly controlled type II diabetic, and has familial hypercholesterolemia. His LAD lesion has been stented twice following his original CABG, but both times he developed in-stent restenosis within a few months. The good news is that his LV function is well preserved. The bad news is he underwent bilateral vein stripping for varicosities in the past. The radial arteries are a consideration, although the right radial was used for cardiac catheterization and cannot be trusted. Unfortunately, upper extremity plethysmography failed to confirm a complete palmar arch on the left, precluding the use of the left radial artery. Now what?

B. Potz
Department of Surgery, Massachusetts General Hospital, Boston, USA
e-mail: bpotz@mgh.harvard.edu

G. Tolis (✉)
Department of Surgery, Brigham and Women's Hospital, Boston, MA, USA
e-mail: gtolis@partners.org

© The Author(s), under exclusive license to Springer Nature Switzerland AG 2022
T. M. Sundt et al. (eds.), *Near Misses in Cardiac Surgery*,
https://doi.org/10.1007/978-3-030-92750-9_22

87

Solution

There is no doubt in your mind that this gentleman needs surgical revascularization, and that long-term patency is a high priority. You have few options for arterial conduit remaining. The right internal thoracic artery (aka right internal mammary artery or RIMA) is the best option, although it raises concerns for wound healing, particularly in an individual with such co-morbidities. You are also concerned that it may not reach the LAD in-situ forcing you to take it as free graft. The midportion of the LAD looks intramyocardial, likely explaining the error made by the earlier surgical team. You remember the admonition never to assume the prior surgeon was incompetent or you may well find yourself in the same tight spot they occupied before you. Aware that anastomosis directly to the aorta can be challenging, you resect a disc of ascending aorta the size of a quarter and patch it with bovine pericardium to which the ITA is easily anastomosed. What seemed rather straightforward initially became quite a bit more complicated!

Discussion

This unfortunate patient suffered a well described complication of coronary bypass operations, the avoidance of which can be particularly challenging in the setting of minimally invasive direct coronary artery bypass grafting in an obese individual. One can easily mistake a large diagonal running parallel to an intramyocardial LAD - or even worse the great cardiac vein - for the intended target. Be that as it may, he needs redo-CABG.

Perhaps the most obvious option, and the one considered first, is the use of the in situ RIMA as his LAD conduit [2]. It may be challenging to reach the LAD depending on the heart size and location of the distal anastomosis as in this case. Skeletonization of the RIMA may provide additional length. The principal disadvantage to using the RIMA in this obese diabetic patient is the increased incidence of sternal wound infection reported in many series comparing bilateral to single ITA strategies, although, again, skeletonizing may reduce this risk [3]. If the RIMA will not reach its target despite skeletonization and removal of all mediastinal fat between the right phrenic nerve and the cavo-innominate junction, the RIMA can be used as a free graft with inflow from the aorta or even as a composite graft from the existing patent LIMA graft [4]. Anastomosis directly to the aorta can be challenging given the discrepancy in vessel wall thickness between the aorta and the ITA, making the hood of a vein graft or a pericardial patch an appealing intermediary.

The radial artery contralateral to the dominant arm is a tempting conduit that spares the blood supply to the sternum [4, 5]. Unfortunately, this patient's Allen Test was positive on the left. In addition, his right radial has been cannulated for cardiac catheterization, an increasingly popular approach but one associated with coronary bypass graft failure [6].

Finally, there have been limited reports of "recycling" the ITA, which might have been possible in this case if sufficient length of ITA were available [7]. This can be accomplished by skeletonizing the existing ITA graft in situ. In years past, cryopreserved saphenous vein was employed on occasion; however, its patency is less than 50% within the first year [8].

References

1. Grau JB, Ferrari G, Mak AW, Shaw RE, Brizzio ME, Mindich BP, Strobeck J, Zapolanski A. Propensity matched analysis of bilateral internal mammary artery versus single left internal mammary artery grafting at 17-year follow-up: validation of a contemporary surgical experience. Eur J Cardiothorac Surg. 2012 Apr;41(4):770–5; discussion 776. doi: https://doi.org/10.1093/ejcts/ezr213. Epub 2012 Jan 20. PMID: 22290908.
2. Gaudino M, Lorusso R, Rahouma M, Abouarab A, Tam DY, Spadaccio C, Saint-Hilary G, Leonard J, Iannaccone M, D'Ascenzo F, Di Franco A, Soletti G, Kamel MK, Lau C, Girardi LN, Schwann TA, Benedetto U, Taggart DP, Fremes SE. Radial artery versus right internal thoracic artery versus saphenous vein as the second conduit for coronary artery bypass surgery: a network meta-analysis of clinical outcomes. J Am Heart Assoc. 2019 Jan 22;8(2): e010839. doi: https://doi.org/10.1161/JAHA.118.010839. PMID: 30636525; PMCID: PMC6497341.
3. Yang JF, Gu CX, Wei H, Liu R, Chen CC, Wang SY, Li B, Hu H, Huang XS. [Off-pump coronary artery bypass grafting with only bilateral internal mammary artery composite Lima-Rima Y graft]. Zhonghua Wai Ke Za Zhi. 2006 Nov 15;44(22):1529-31. Chinese. PMID: 17359655.
4. Grau JB, Johnson CK, Kuschner CE, Ferrari G, Shaw RE, Brizzio ME, Zapolanski A. Impact of pump status and conduit choice in coronary artery bypass: A 15-year follow-up study in 1412 propensity-matched patients. J Thorac Cardiovasc Surg. 2015 Apr;149(4):1027-33.e2. doi: https://doi.org/10.1016/j.jtcvs.2014.12.031. Epub 2014 Dec 20. PMID: 25648476.
5. Chwann TA, Hashim SW, Badour S, Obeid M, Engoren M, Tranbaugh RF, Bonnell MR, Habib RH. Equipoise between radial artery and right internal thoracic artery as the second arterial conduit in left internal thoracic artery-based coronary artery bypass graft surgery: a multi-institutional study. Eur J Cardiothorac Surg. 2016 Jan;49(1):188-95. doi: https://doi.org/10.1093/ejcts/ezv093. Epub 2015 Mar 11. PMID: 25762396.
6. Mounsey CA, Mawhinney JA, Werner RS, Taggart DP. Does Previous Transradial Catheterization Preclude Use of the Radial Artery as a Conduit in Coronary Artery Bypass Surgery? Circulation. 2016 Aug 30;134(9):681-8. doi: https://doi.org/10.1161/CIRCULATIONAHA.116.022992. PMID: 27572880 Review.
7. El Oumeiri B, Glineur D, Price J, Boodhwani M, Etienne PY, Poncelet A, De Kerchove L, Papadatos S, Noirhomme P, El Khoury G. Recycling of internal thoracic arteries in reoperative coronary surgery: in-hospital and midterm results. Ann Thorac Surg. 2011 Apr;91(4):1165-8. doi: https://doi.org/10.1016/j.athoracsur.2010.11.073. PMID: 21440139.
8. Laub W, Muralidharan S, Clancy Eldredge J, Chen C, Adkins MS, Fernandez J, Anderson W, McGrath LB. Cryopreserved allograft veins as alternative coronary artery bypass conduits: Early phase results The Annals of Thoracic Surgery. 1992 Nov;54(5):826–83.

Chapter 23
Intraoperative Coagulopathy

Monica Miller and Michael G. Fitzsimons

Problem

The morning started like any other. The day was sure to be busy because you are supervising a resident in two back-to-back cases and you are also the lead cardiac anesthesiologist responsible for overseeing the daily workflow for the service. Your first case is a 68-year-old male with triple vessel coronary artery disease and normal heart function scheduled to undergo coronary artery bypass grafting. This is your resident's second rotation through cardiac, so you're hopeful this "normal EF CABG" will be a straightforward case for him. Induction and line placement go very smoothly. The surgical fellow quickly takes down the left IMA, setting a personal record. The patient transitions on and off cardiopulmonary bypass without any difficulty. After evaluating the grafts, the surgeon asks for the radio to be turned to their favorite 80's rock station with the volume turned up. She directs your resident to give protamine and you step out to deal with administrative duties. It seems you have only been gone for a few minutes when you get a call from your resident—the surgeon is frustrated because of ongoing bleeding. The radio is now off—a bad sign—and the surgeon is asking about the coagulation studies and none too nicely. A messy end to what seemed a perfectly smooth case. Your resident hung platelets and FFP which seemed only to upset the surgeon more—the patient's preoperative hematocrit was 41% and up to now he has received no blood products. Hurling yourself into the breech, you speak up asking the surgeon what's wrong only to be confronted with a brusque "does the field look wet to you?" You ask the resident to run another ACT and hurry back. Things seemed to be going so well. What a way to start the day. The result of the ACT is 453 s.

M. Miller · M. G. Fitzsimons (✉)
Division of Cardiac Anesthesia, Department of Anesthesia, Critical Care, and Pain Medicine,
Massachusetts General Hospital, 55 Fruit Street, Boston, MA 02114, USA
e-mail: Mfitzsimons@mgh.harvard.edu

© The Author(s), under exclusive license to Springer Nature Switzerland AG 2022
T. M. Sundt et al. (eds.), *Near Misses in Cardiac Surgery*,
https://doi.org/10.1007/978-3-030-92750-9_23

Solution

As you look at the anesthesia workstation, the problem at hand becomes evident. Sherlock Holmes has nothing on you! Vials of heparin and protamine, which are similar in appearance, lie side by side on the workstation. Upon further inspection you identify that the protamine vial is unopened while a half-full vial of heparin is on the anesthesia tray. You ask the resident about your observation who then acknowledges he may have inadvertently administered additional heparin instead of protamine. You notify the surgeon immediately and proceed with protamine administration. The bleeding improves, a repeat ACT is 120 s, and everyone relaxes. Not a disaster, just a near miss.

Discussion

Medication errors in anesthesia, often referred to as adverse drug events (ADEs) or adverse drug reactions (ADRs), include administration of the wrong drug, dose, concentration, repetition of administration or omission of critical administration. The incidence may exceed 5%, These errors can lead to potential life-threatening adverse events. Literature on this topic is limited and largely driven by self-reporting, thus underrepresenting the true incidence. Various factors contribute to error including distraction, inattention, haste, lack of familiarity or experience with a medication, and lack of communication. Similarities in medication packaging and labeling have also been identified as potential causes. Certain drugs may look alike-sound alike (LASA). New technologies are in place including bar-code assisted medication systems which have improved safety outside the operating room and demonstrate promise intraoperatively.

In this case, inadvertent heparin administration led to ongoing coagulopathy and bleeding, noticed by the surgeon, despite a directive to administer protamine. The team appropriately performed repeat analysis and a review of the processes (checking medication vials) which raised the suspicion of medication error. Although the patient remained hemodynamically stable, transfusion and the associated risks may have been avoided had protamine been correctly administered. This incident did not result in injury, but there was a potential for harm.

The definition of what constitutes harm often prompts the conversation of whether patient disclosure of error is warranted. Most would agree errors leading to serious adverse events or outcomes must be disclosed. There is less consensus among providers when errors pose a potential for harm. Apprehension regarding disclosure is often related to fears of subsequent patient mistrust and litigation, yet research has shown the opposite is true. Transparency and immediate disclosure will foster the patient-physician relationship and may provide valuable information that prompts process improvement to prevent similar errors from recurring. Transparency in turn depend upon the existence of a safe culture within the operating room that allows disclosure without shame. This is the key to establishing a learning environment that optimizes team performance, making the team even more than resilient. It is anti-fragile!

Bibliography

1. Webster CS, Merry AF, Larsson L, McGrath KA, Weller J. The frequency and nature of drug administration error during anaesthesia. Anaesth Intensive Care. 2001;29:494e500.
2. Nanji KC, Shaikh S, Seger DL, Bates DW. Evaluation of perioperative medication errors and adverse drug events. Anesthesiology. 2016;124:25–34.
3. Beverley A Orser, David U, Michael R Cohen; Perioperative Medication Errors: Building Safer Systems. Anesthesiology. 2016;124:1–3.
4. Chamberlain CJ, Koniaris LG, Wu AW, Pawlik TM. Disclosure of "Nonharmful" medical errors and other events: duty to disclose. Arch Surg. 2012;147(3):282–6.
5. Cooper RL, Fogarty-Mack P, Kroll HR, Barach P. Medication safety in Anesthesia: epidemiology, causes, and lessons learned in achieving reliable patient outcomes. Inn Anesthes Clin. 2019;57:78–95.

Chapter 24
Hypoxia after Atrial Septal Defect (ASD) Closure

Jordan P. Bloom and Duke E. Cameron

Problem

A 25-year-old woman with an ostium secundum atrial septal defect (ASD) undergoes autologous pericardial patch closure of the defect via a right anterior thoracotomy. A double lumen endotracheal tube has been placed, and cardiopulmonary bypass is conducted via femoral arterial, femoral venous, and superior vena cava cannulation through the right atrium. Fibrillatory arrest is used to prevent air embolism. On separation from cardiopulmonary bypass, there is profound systemic arterial desaturation. Your anesthesiologist confirms there is good air entry into both lungs and bronchoscopy is unremarkable. TEE shows preserved biventricular function and there are no leaks seen around the ASD patch but there are color flow patterns near the IVC that are puzzling.

What has happened and how will you proceed?

Solution

The inferior margin of the ASD patch was inadvertently sewn to the Eustachian valve rather than the inferior rim of the atrial septal defect, effectively baffling IVC flow to the left atrium and creating a large right-to-left shunt and hypoxia. The thoracotomy approach and snaring of the IVC may obscure the true ASD margin. Although it is important to rule out pulmonary causes of de-saturation,

J. P. Bloom · D. E. Cameron (✉)
Department of Surgery, Massachusetts General Hospital, Boston, MA, USA
e-mail: decameron@mgh.harvard.edu

J. P. Bloom
e-mail: jpbloom@mgh.harvard.edu

© The Author(s), under exclusive license to Springer Nature Switzerland AG 2022   95
T. M. Sundt et al. (eds.), *Near Misses in Cardiac Surgery*,
https://doi.org/10.1007/978-3-030-92750-9_24

such as contralateral lung collapse or bronchial plugging, this technical error should be kept in mind whenever there is hypoxia after ASD closure. Simple peri-patch leaks do not lead to desaturation because the result is a residual left-to-right shunt, but a dehisced or malpositioned patch may obstruct venous return and direct caval flow to the left atrium. In this case, the right atrium must be re-opened and the patch revised.

Discussion

Atrial septal defect is the second most common congenital lesion in adults after bicuspid aortic valve [1]. Patients are often asymptomatic until adulthood. Potential complications of untreated ASD include atrial arrhythmias, paradoxical embolization, cerebral abscess, right ventricular failure and tricuspid regurgitation, and pulmonary hypertension that may become irreversible and lead to right-to-left shunting (Eisenmenger syndrome). Small ASDs (<8 mm) in asymptomatic patients may not require closure.

The traditional approach for surgical repair of an ASD has been via median sternotomy. In the modern era, minimally invasive and robotic approaches are becoming more common [2]. Many surgeons recite the adage "Never compromise on exposure." This case highlights that even a "simple" procedure can become complicated, particularly when exposure is limited. Pericardial or prosthetic patch closure is generally the treatment of choice for open repair of a secundum ASD. Surgical closure can be performed with <1% mortality and preservation of normal life expectancy [3]. Percutaneous devices for ASD closure exist and two are FDA approved; the ideal lesion for percutaneous closure is a secundum defect ≤ 38 mm in diameter with a rim of tissue around the defect of at least 5 mm [4]. Patients for percutaneous closure should not have pulmonary hypertension or diastolic dysfunction, and the presence of concomitant structural heart disease, such as partial anomalous venous return, should be ruled out. Observational studies have reported similar safety and efficacy for open and transcatheter closure.

It is critical to know and identify relevant anatomic structures when performing patch closure of an intracardiac defect or using a patch to baffle blood flow. This is a common challenge in congenital heart surgery. In this case, the key to successful repair is to identify the true inferior margin of the ASD and secure the patch to this margin. With vacuum assist on the IVC cannula, the caval snare can be released and the Eustachian valve identified and even resected if necessary. In some scenarios, it may be safer to arrest the heart and use moderate systemic hypothermia.

References

1. Ntiloudi D, Giannakoulas G, Parcharidou D, Panagiotidis T, Gatzoulis MA, Karvounis H. Adult congenital heart disease: A paradigm of epidemiological change. Vol. 218, Int Journa of Cardiology. Elsevier Ireland Ltd; 2016. pp. 269–74.
2. Butera G, Biondi-Zoccai G, Sangiorgi G, Abella R, Giamberti A, Bussadori C, et al. Percutaneous versus surgical closure of secundum atrial septal defects: A systematic review and meta-analysis of currently available clinical evidence [Internet]. Vol. 7, EuroIntervention. EuroIntervention; 2011. pp. 377–85.
3. Hopkins RA, Bert AA, Buchholz B, Guarino K, Meyers M. Surgical patch closure of atrial septal defects. Ann Thorac Surg. 2004;77(6):2144–9.
4. Prokšelj K, Koželj M, Zadnik V, Podnar T. Echocardiographic characteristics of secundum-type atrial septal defects in adult patients: Implications for percutaneous closure using amplatzer septal occluders. J Am Soc Echocardiogr. 2004;17(11):1167–72.

Chapter 25
Intraoperative Pulmonary Hemorrhage

Lynze R. Franko and Kenneth T. Shelton

Problem

Another day at the office. Your first case is a 72-year-old hypertensive patient with severe triple-vessel coronary artery disease and an EF of 35% who will undergo three vessel coronary artery bypass grafting. Prior to induction of anesthesia, the anesthesia team inserts a Swan-Ganz pulmonary artery catheter and records right atrial, pulmonary artery, and pulmonary capillary wedge pressures of 10, 33/19, and 15 mmHg, respectively. You take down the internal thoracic artery, while your physician assistant harvests saphenous vein endoscopically. Good conduit! You ask for heparin and cannulate for bypass when the ACT rises above baseline. As the perfusionist runs the pre-bypass checklist, the anesthesiologist informs you that dark blood has suddenly flooded the endotracheal tube. You are incredulous. This has arisen at an extremely awkward moment in a heparinized, cannulated patient whose conduit has already been harvested! And now the oxygen saturations are falling. What to do?

Solution

You suspect the Swan-Ganz catheter has perforated the pulmonary artery, probably on the right side since most pulmonary artery catheters flow to that side; therefore, increasing the risk of right-sided artery perforation [1]. Upon opening the right

L. R. Franko
Department of Surgery, Massachusetts General Hospital, Boston, MA, USA
e-mail: lfranko@mgh.harvard.edu

K. T. Shelton (✉)
Department of Anesthesia, Massachusetts General Hospital, Boston, MA, USA
e-mail: Kshelton@mgh.harvard.edu

© The Author(s), under exclusive license to Springer Nature Switzerland AG 2022
T. M. Sundt et al. (eds.), *Near Misses in Cardiac Surgery*,
https://doi.org/10.1007/978-3-030-92750-9_25

99

mediastinal pleura, you identify a diffuse subpleural hemorrhage in the lateral basal segment of the right lower lobe. You decide to proceed with the operation as planned because the patient's coronary artery disease is severe and once cardiopulmonary bypass has begun there should be near-total decompression of the pulmonary circulation with a concomitant reduction in the hemoptysis. Should a pulmonary procedure be required subsequently, it could be performed more safely in a revascularized patient. A bronchial blocker is placed by the anesthesia team. The coronary bypass operation proceeds uneventfully. Prior to separating the patient from cardiopulmonary bypass, the anesthesiologist places a double lumen endotracheal tube, performs bronchoscopy with a pediatric fiberoptic scope, and suctions the right mainstem bronchus. You successfully wean from bypass and administer protamine. The timing is particularly risky given the restoration of pulmonary artery blood flow. Much to your relief, there is no change in the size of the subpleural hematoma, although you know you must continue to be vigilant because of the high risk of life-threatening recurrent hemorrhage [1].

Discussion

Of the "birds of the thoracic cage" (esopha-goose, va-goose, thoracic duck, azy-goose and swan), the Swan may be the most dangerous. This patient has experienced one of numerous potential complications associated with placing pulmonary artery catheters at the beginning of a cardiac surgical procedure. In this instance, a peripheral pulmonary artery was ruptured by a pulmonary artery catheter. In one study, this complication was found in approximately 0.1% of cases with a hospital mortality rate of 42% [1]. Although this may occur in patients with pulmonary hypertension and fragile pulmonary vasculature, more often it results from a miscalculation of the length of catheter required for wedging in an individual patient or from overzealous insertion technique. Pulmonary artery perforations can be prevented by using only gentle pressure on insertion and by not advancing farther than the right atrium with the balloon deflated. Once in place, the balloon should be inflated slowly, with just enough air to initiate a wedge tracing and no more. Preferably, the catheter should always be withdrawn a few centimeters before inflating the balloon and then advanced with the balloon inflated into a wedge position. The catheter should never be withdrawn with the balloon inflated. In the patient with pulmonary hypertension, measurements of wedge pressure should probably be avoided as much as possible. Patients over 65 years old also have an increased risk of perforation [1]. The pulmonary artery catheter should be withdrawn to the main pulmonary artery routinely after the initiation of cardiopulmonary bypass to prevent a catheter stiffened by hypothermia from perforating the pulmonary artery when the heart is elevated from the pericardium for exposure during surgery.

Once catheter-induced hemoptysis has been identified, maintaining gas exchange is critical. Positive end expiratory pressure and interventions to reduce pulmonary artery pressure may effectively control lesser degrees of bleeding. Treatment also includes placement of a bronchial blocker initially to obtain immediate isolation and prevent flooding of the opposite mainstem bronchus if the bleeding persists. Subsequently, this can be transitioned to a double lumen endotracheal tube. The benefits of a double lumen endotracheal tube are: it allows direct visualization, suctioning and possible intervention, and it provides the ability to safely ventilate each lung separately long term if required [2]. One treatment option after confirmatory angiogram may include selective embolization to reduce the likelihood of recurrence or pseudoaneurysm formation [1–3]. If the patient is hemodynamically unstable, if the vessel injury is proximal, or if the bleeding is extensive, surgical repair via vessel reconstruction, lobectomy, or pulmonary resection is recommended [1]. If the parenchymal hemorrhage occupies a majority of the lobe, pulmonary resection may be required, although surgical intervention has been associated with greater mortality [1], likely due to the greater severity of injury requiring such intervention. An alternative to pulmonary resection in a patient with poor pulmonary reserve is to try to support the patient on ECMO during the acute phase of hypoxia [1, 3]. If bleeding becomes problematic during the course of surgery, the right pulmonary artery can be clamped intrapericardially between the superior vena cava and the aorta for temporary control.

Other significant problems associated with central vascular access during preparation for surgery include accidental puncture or even cannulation of the carotid artery with an introducer sheath. Should this occur in a patient who needs an immediate procedure requiring heparinization, the sheath should be removed, and the carotid injury repaired with sutures under direct vision. It is also possible to advance a central line catheter through the posterior wall of the innominate vein into the pleural space, an error that may only become apparent when drugs administered centrally fail to have effect. This injury can be repaired under direct vision (with difficulty) after opening the pleural space.

The risk of serious complications associated with pulmonary artery catheters is less than 1% [1, 4]. Additional complications include right ventricular rupture, catheter coiling/knotting in the right ventricle, accidental suturing of the catheter during cardiac surgery, and heart block [1, 4]. Right ventricular wall rupture can be repaired intraoperatively or monitored conservatively depending on the patient's hemodynamics. Another potential complication of Swan-Ganz catheterization is induction of a right bundle branch [5]. Should a pulmonary artery catheter be required in a patient with persistent left bundle branch block, external pacing pads and a pulmonary artery catheter with a port for introducing the pacing electrode should be employed. This is particularly true if the left bundle branch block is new as the risk for developing complete heart block is higher [5].

Learning Objectives

(1) Understand high risk PA catheter placement (older patients, cold patients, over wedging, careful inflation)
(2) Understand heart block concerns (Patient with pre-existing left bundle branch block (LBBB), need for transcutaneous pacing, transvenous pacing, etc.)
(3) Understand management [bronchial blocker, double lumen tube (DLT), operative management]

References

1. Sirivella S, Gielchinsky I, Parsonnet V. Management of catheter-induced pulmonary artery perforation: a rare complication in cardiovascular operations. Ann Thorac Surg. 2001;72 (6):2056–9.
2. Awad H, et al. Bronchial blocker versus double-lumen tube for lung isolation with massive hemoptysis during cardiac surgery. J Cardiothorac Vasc Anesth. 2013;27(3):e26–8.
3. Rudziński PN et al. Pulmonary artery rupture as a complication of Swan-Ganz catheter application. Diagnosis and endovascular treatment: a single centre's experience. Postepy w kardiologii interwencyjnej. Adv Interv Cardiol. 2016;12(2):135–9.
4. Bossert T, et al. Swan-Ganz catheter-induced severe complications in cardiac surgery: right ventricular perforation, knotting, and rupture of a pulmonary artery. J Card Surg. 2006;21 (3):292–5.
5. Morris D, Mulvihill D, Lew WY. Risk of developing complete heart block during bedside pulmonary artery catheterization in patients with left bundle-branch block. Arch Intern Med. 1987;147(11):2005–10.

Chapter 26
Femoral Arterial Cannulation

Thoralf Sundt

Problem

Your colleague in the division of general thoracic surgery has taken on a particularly challenging case. The patient is a 62-year-old woman with limited pulmonary reserve and a very proximal but localized carcinoma of the left upper lobe. The plan is to do a bronchial and pulmonary artery sleeve resection but the team has lost control of the proximal pulmonary artery (PA) and now find themselves with uncontrollable bleeding. You have been summoned to the operating room to get the patient on pump so the situation can be rescued. When you arrive, the staff has a finger in the PA and the fellow has exposed the left common femoral artery and vein. The pump has just been set up in the corner of the room and the perfusionists are in the process of priming. You ask for heparin to be given as you scrub your hands.

The femoral vein is of adequate caliber, and you place a pursestring suture in the ventral surface. The artery is a bit more problematic, with calcification posteriorly but an adequate pulse. Again, a pursestring suture and you are ready to go. The ACT is therapeutic. You pass the venous cannula without resistance over a wire after the anesthesiologist confirms its presence in the right atrium. You then pass the arterial wire into the aorta via the femoral artery, again with confirmation from the anesthesiologist by echo, but as you insert the 18 Fr cannula, you meet some resistance and stop. The cannula is already several centimeters into the artery and you do not want to elevate a plaque. The wire is removed, the connection to the pump is made, and bypass is initiated. Flow seems adequate to start, but the anesthesiologist reports that despite escalating levophed the radial pressure is persistently low. The perfusionist tells you the line pressure is high despite the low systemic pressure. You reach inside the chest and feel the descending thoracic

T. Sundt (✉)
Chief, Division of Cardiac Surgery, Massachusetts General Hospital, Boston, MA, USA
e-mail: tsundt@mgh.harvard.edu

© The Author(s), under exclusive license to Springer Nature Switzerland AG 2022   103
T. M. Sundt et al. (eds.), *Near Misses in Cardiac Surgery*,
https://doi.org/10.1007/978-3-030-92750-9_26

aorta. The aorta looks normal but is as tight as a drum. The anesthesiologists do not see a dissection flap in the descending thoracic aorta. As you struggle to make sense of the situation, you realize you could have simply cannulated the descending thoracic aorta for arterial return! Just then the anesthesiologist tells you they see a dissection flap in the ascending aorta.

What in the world is going on? And what to do?

Solution

At this point your options are limited. This is likely a retrograde dissection and there is no utility in cannulating the descending thoracic aorta directly because there is no true lumen. The retrograde dissection has compressed the true lumen entirely, and for this reason no flap was apparent by echo. Axillary cannulation is impractical. The only real cannulation option is transapical. You open the pericardium, place a pledgeted pursestring suture in the apex of the left ventricle, and pass an arterial inflow cannula via the apex across the aortic valve and into the ascending aorta. As you stop the pump and leave blood in the heart, the anesthesiologists inform you that the cerebral oximetry has fallen dramatically and the SedLine processed EEG is severely depressed. Just as you transfer arterial inflow to the apical cannula, the heart fibrillates. Despite application of internal paddles, the patient cannot be defibrillated. You suspect the dissection has extended proximally to the coronary arteries. In conversation with your thoracic surgical colleague you determine the situation is, for all practical purposes, unrecoverable. It was a long shot for a patient with limited pulmonary reserve. Your best judgment is that the most prudent course of action is to withdraw therapy. This one was not just a Near Miss.

Discussion

In this instance the femoral arterial cannula has indeed caused a retrograde dissection. You felt reassured initially because you did it by the book, passing the cannula over a wire and not forcing it. True, it did not advance as far as you would have liked, i.e., into the iliac, but in the early years of cardiac surgery and common use of the femoral artery for cardiopulmonary bypass, femoral arterial cannulae were only inserted a few centimeters into the common femoral artery. There must have been a susceptible plaque which, on initiation of bypass, elevated and caused the dissection. The patient's aorta is sufficiently atherosclerotic that the descending aorta did not discolor suggesting dissection. The echo was deceptive because all the flow went into the false lumen. There was no flap. It was only when the flap appeared in the ascending aorta that the diagnosis was confirmed. Worse, once the dissection occurred there were few options for recovery.

This is an example of the best therapy being prevention. Palpable atherosclerotic disease of the femoral artery raised concerns and when the cannula would not pass easily, a different course of action might have been undertaken. The bleeding from the pulmonary artery was under control, and as is so often the case, the most important thing you could have done was stop and think. There was already a momentum to cannulate the femoral artery because your colleagues had exposed it and laid it out for you on a silver platter. But the entire descending thoracic aorta was accessible to you via the left thoracotomy and it would have been far simpler to cannulate that initially, or, with resistance felt in passing the femoral cannula, to change course. All this before flow was initiated and dissection occurred.

An additional point to be made in this case is the impact of tunnel vision and cognitive confirmation bias. In the moment, you could not make sense of the situation because the aorta did not look grossly dissected and the echocardiographer did not see a flap. However, all other signs pointed to intraoperative dissection – a drop in radial artery pressure and high line pressures on the pump with a tense descending thoracic aorta after a problematic arterial cannulation. It was only the echo images that did not fit the diagnosis. If they had been rejected, the patient could have been promptly weaned from bypass, restoring antegrade flow in the descending thoracic aorta, and the dissection might have been reversed before it extended proximally to the aortic root. The risk of falling victim to these cognitive biases is made worse by time pressure, a ubiquitous aspect of our specialty. Under these circumstances, humans rely on fast, intuitive thinking and on pattern recognition. But when things don't make sense, we must make a conscious effort to switch our thinking to slow algorithmic thinking: list all of the facts, all the possible explanations, and all of the procedural options. Easier said than done.

Bibliography

1. Kahneman D. Thinking fast and slow. 2011. New York. Farrar, Straus and Giroux.
2. Klein GA. Sources of power: how people make decisions. Cambridge, Mass: MIT Press; 1998. p. 1–30.

Chapter 27
Hypoxia on ECMO

Jerome C. Crowley

Problem

You are covering the cardiac surgical service over a holiday weekend for your colleagues, and you begin your morning by making rounds on the ICU patients. One of the first patients you see is your colleagues' patient who was placed on peripheral ECMO because of inability to separate from cardiopulmonary bypass with a post-operative course complicated by significant bleeding. The bedside nurse happily informs you that the bleeding has almost completely resolved based on chest tube output and laboratory markers and you breathe a sigh of relief at not having to perform a chest exploration on a holiday weekend. Upon further review of the patient's vitals, you are also pleased to note that the patient's pulsatility has improved with the bedside echocardiogram performed by the intensivist suggesting myocardial recovery. Intravenous calcium channel blockers are being infused for hypertension. The only red flag is an oxygen saturation of 90% despite what should be adequate ECMO support. You note that the arterial line is in the left femoral artery. You request a right radial arterial line be placed and a blood gas taken.

While making rounds on the wards you are paged with the results of the arterial blood gas; the patient is not acidotic, but the right radial arterial line shows an arterial oxygen saturation of only 87%. The ECMO specialists at the bedside check pre- and post-membrane gases which reveal a well-functioning oxygenator. You return to the bedside where the right-hand saturation is now reading 84% despite 100% delivered oxygen on the ventilator and on the ECMO circuit.

STAT chest X-ray reveals what you fear, severe pulmonary edema related to the massive transfusion the patient received in the past 48 h. You request aggressive diuresis but to your dismay minimal response is noted to loop diuretics because of significant acute kidney injury sustained during the surgery. Nephrology is urgently

J. C. Crowley (✉)
Department of Anesthesia, Massachusetts General Hospital, Boston, MA, USA
e-mail: jccrowley@mgh.harvard.edu

© The Author(s), under exclusive license to Springer Nature Switzerland AG 2022   107
T. M. Sundt et al. (eds.), *Near Misses in Cardiac Surgery*,
https://doi.org/10.1007/978-3-030-92750-9_27

consulted, and continuous dialysis is begun but now the arterial saturation has fallen to 78%. The respiratory therapist has increased the ventilator settings to attempt to rectify the situation but you worry the high airway pressures will further injure the lungs. There is some brief discussion about possible shunting from the intravenous calcium channel blockers, but the progression of the hypoxia is forcing your hand. You sigh in frustration for having to deal with an unstable patient that isn't even your own as you re-activate the ECMO team for circuit re-configuration.

Solution

After arrival of the ECMO team and placement of a TEE probe, you prepare for re-configuration to veno-arterial-venous (V-AV) ECMO. Using an ultrasound and Seldinger technique, you place an appropriately sized arterial cannula in the right internal jugular vein and withdraw the femoral venous cannula to the level of the proximal inferior vena cava under TEE guidance. Next, after pausing the ECMO circuit briefly, you Y-connect the internal jugular cannula with the femoral arterial cannula. After re-initiating support with the new hybrid configuration, you note an improvement in oxygen saturation and a decrease in mean arterial blood pressure.

You request the cessation of vasodilators and, using adjustable clamps, control the flow to roughly 2 LPM down the femoral arterial cannula and 4 LPM flowing from the venous cannula. However, there is now substantial chatter noted on the femoral venous line, and based on the pulmonary edema, additional volume is not likely to further the patient's clinical progress. You next prepare the contralateral groin and place an additional femoral venous cannula to aid drainage. After Y-connecting this cannula to the other femoral venous cannula, you are able to flow appropriately without chatter. Chest X-ray confirms appropriate cannula position and repeat arterial blood gases now show a saturation of 99%. You instruct the intensive care team to continue with volume removal as tolerated and book the patient for arterial cannula decannulation in the operating room the following day.

Discussion

This patient is displaying the classic findings of differential hypoxia, also known as Harlequin or North–South Syndrome. This is caused by the nature of the flow of blood on peripheral femoral VA ECMO. Oxygenated blood flows retrograde from the femoral artery where it mixes with blood being ejected from the native heart. When native cardiac function is poor, the mixing likely occurs very close to the aortic valve and systemic oxygenation is maintained. This is monitored by always checking blood gas measurements and peripheral saturations from the right upper extremity as this is most likely to correlate with carotid blood oxygenation. (It should be noted that the oxygen saturation of the blood perfusing the coronaries is never known). As myocardial function recovers (or if a percutaneous ventricular assist device is in place and support from the VAD is increased) the mixing of blood from the native cardiac output and the ECMO circuit moves further down the aorta. If native lung function is intact (pure cardiac failure) this is likely of little consequence as the native ejection is also likely well oxygenated. However, if the patient has significant pulmonary disease (common in patients with volume overload or acute respiratory distress syndrome) then the native cardiac output will be significantly hypoxic. This means the brain is receiving predominantly hypoxic blood.

Management can take several approaches depending on the patient's condition. ECMO circuit function should be verified to make sure appropriate oxygenation is occurring in the circuit. Native cardiac function should be assessed via pulsatility and echocardiography if possible. The first maneuver should be to optimize ventilator settings, but in the setting of severe ARDS this may not be enough. A second maneuver would be to convert the patient to central cannulation which will avoid the mixing problem; however, in a patient with recovering cardiac function this may represent a step back in recovery as it requires a sternotomy and potentially an open chest. The solution described here is to convert the patient's ECMO circuit to a hybrid configuration, V-AV ECMO.

V-AV ECMO can be thought of as a combination of both venovenous and venoarterial ECMO. Blood is drained from the patient and oxygenated. Then part of the blood is returned to the femoral artery to support the blood pressure/perfusion (veno-arterial component) and part is returned to the internal jugular vein to "pre-oxygenate" the blood prior to circulating through the lungs (veno-venous component). The relative proportion of flow to each can be titrated to the mean arterial pressure and the right upper extremity oxygen saturation. Once the arterial limb is sufficiently down-titrated, the patient is likely ready for removal of the arterial component and can continue on veno-venous ECMO until the lungs recover. It is important to note that V-AV ECMO requires higher flows and therefore additional venous drainage may be needed (effectively creating a VV-AV ECMO circuit).

Bibliography

1. Sidebotham D. Troubleshooting adult ECMO. J Extra Corpor Technol. 2011 Mar;43(1): P27-32. PMID: 21449237.
2. Biscotti M, Lee A, Basner RC, Agerstrand C, Abrams D, Brodie D, Bacchetta M. Hybrid configurations via percutaneous access for extracorporeal membrane oxygenation: a single-center experience. ASAIO J. 2014 Nov-Dec;60(6):635–42
3. Brasseur A, Scolletta S, Lorusso R, Taccone FS. Hybrid extracorporeal membrane oxygenation. J Thorac Dis. 2018 Mar;10(Suppl 5):S707–15.
4. Eckman PM, Katz JN, El Banayosy A, Bohula EA, Sun B, van Diepen S. Veno-arterial extracorporeal membrane oxygenation for cardiogenic shock: an introduction for the busy clinician. Circulation. 2019 Dec 10;140(24):2019–37.

Chapter 28
Laser Lead Extraction

Travis Hull and Masaki Funamoto

Problem

You have been working hard to establish a close working relationship with your colleagues in cardiac electrophysiology (EP) as they build a lead extraction program. While "standing by" for them is less than your idea of fun, you have seen the catastrophic consequences when lead extractions go wrong outside the operating room. And who knows, there may even be an avenue for them to help you build your surgical arrhythmia practice! Relationships with colleagues are important.

This morning they have asked you to assist in the removal of a single chamber pacemaker in an 84-year-old gentleman with sick sinus syndrome who presented 2 days ago with fevers, altered mental status, and *Staphylococcus aureus* bacteremia. Transesophageal echocardiography (TEE) shows a 1.3 × 2 cm mobile echodensity consistent with vegetation on the atrial portion of his pacer lead, normal cardiac function, and no pericardial effusion. The pacemaker was placed via a transvenous left subclavian vein percutaneous approach over 20 years ago, increasing the likelihood that laser lead extraction will be necessary.

You prepped from chin to knees, with cardiac perfusion and the instruments for sternotomy and cannulation on standby. After removing the generator, you mobilize the leads down to the anchoring cuff and step aside for the cardiologists from EP to perform the lead extraction with laser. Suspecting that the laser lead explant will take some time, you dash to the OR lounge to grab a coffee until it's your turn to come back and close the pacer pocket. You nearly choke on the first sip of your $8 soy latte as you toss it in the trash and run to the operating room after receiving a STAT page from the circulating nurse. The patient has become hemodynamically

T. Hull
Department of Surgery, Massachusetts General Hospital, Boston, MA, USA
e-mail: Thull1@partners.org

M. Funamoto (✉)
Department of Cardiothoracic Surgery, Methodist Hospital, San Antonio, USA

© The Author(s), under exclusive license to Springer Nature Switzerland AG 2022   111
T. M. Sundt et al. (eds.), *Near Misses in Cardiac Surgery*,
https://doi.org/10.1007/978-3-030-92750-9_28

unstable with a rising CVP and falling SBP. You burst into the operating room and see the TEE images that confirm your suspicion; a large pericardial effusion that wasn't present pre-operatively. The right atrium (RA) is collapsed, and the interventricular septum is bowed into the left ventricle (LV).

Solution

Based on the patient's hemodynamics and TEE data, you quickly realize that the patient has developed cardiac tamponade from a perforation created on attempted extraction of the chronically indwelling, infected pacer lead. As you head for the scrub sink you hear the cardiologist calling out over his shoulder to see if you think percutaneous drainage might get the job done without sternotomy. Unfortunately, your limited but profoundly memorable experience with these cases tells you that a hemodynamic collapse of this magnitude is more than likely due to a tear in the SVC or even an RV perforation; an attempt at catheter drainage only risks further delay. You proceed with a subxyphoid pericardial window, as it is a more reliable option for drainage of the large pericardial effusion that likely contains a component of clot and can easily be extended to a full sternotomy if necessary. You make an 8 cm subxyphoid incision and dissect through the subcutaneous tissue until the pericardium is visualized. When you open it, a brisk gush of dark red blood and clot is evacuated, and the patient's hemodynamics quickly improve. You insert the suction device into the pericardium and note that copious amounts of blood continue to drain, and the patient becomes hypotensive despite aggressive fluid resuscitation with a heart rate in the 130 s.

The perfusionist, your partner in all such disasters, has been paying close attention and without a word from you is already priming the pump even as the anesthesia team initiates the massive transfusion protocol via a rapid infuser. You open the sternum and enter the pericardium. There is dark red blood rapidly welling up from the right side of the heart from a laceration of the superior vena cava (SVC) at the SVC to right atrial (RA) junction that extends posteriorly along the lateral wall. At that moment, the patient becomes unstable hemodynamically. You ask anesthesia to heparinize the patient and quickly insert a 21 Fr cannula into the ascending aorta without a purse string. You initiate bypass, temporarily using a Poole suction for venous return until you can insert a 29/37 Fr dual stage cannula into the RA appendage. You then place the Poole suction into the laceration in the SVC.

You are now able to achieve full flow on cardiopulmonary bypass (CPB) and both the patient and you are stable. You remove the pacer lead without further issue and close the tract in the pocket where the lead entered the left subclavian vein. You turn your attention to repairing the SVC laceration. You consider your options: primary repair or patch repair? Despite your eagerness to close the hole, you have seen too many cases of SVC syndrome, a notoriously difficult surgical challenge. Instead, you decide that bicaval cannulation will allow for better visualization and patch repair of the posterior aspect of the large irregular laceration. The patient is stable, and you need to get this repair right. You place a 24 Fr right angled cannula above the tear and replace the dual stage cannula with a 28 Fr single stage cannula in the inferior vena cava (IVC) so that a snare can be placed if necessary. After a quick exchange of venous return cannulae you repair the defect with a generous autologous pericardial patch using a 4–0 running Prolene suture. You wean off bypass uneventfully and hemostasis is excellent after protamine administration. You close the chest, and the patient is sent to the intensive care unit, where he has an uneventful recovery and is discharge on post-operative day 5.

Discussion

In the contemporary setting, permanent pacemaker (PPM) and implantable cardioverter-defibrillator (ICD) extraction has become a collaboration between EP and cardiac surgery. While EP is usually able to remove pacer leads without complication or the assistance of a surgeon, the risk of perforation of the subclavian vein, innominate vein, SVC, RA, or right ventricle (RV) is not negligible, with an incidence of approximately 0.14–0.8% [1, 2]. Thus, it is essential to identify patients at risk for perforation and prepare accordingly. This includes performing these procedures in a hybrid cardiac surgery OR, adequate exposure by prepping and draping the patient from chin to chest, open cardiac surgery tools and CPB on standby, and a pre-operative discussion with cardiac anesthesia regarding the need for intra-operative TEE and pre- or intra-operative placement of monitoring (arterial) or resuscitative (central venous) lines, especially in high risk or frail patients. Patient risk factors for perforation include older age, female sex, left bundle-branch block, heart failure, and non-single chamber devices [1]. Additional risk factors for perforation during PPM/ICD explanation include the indication for explant (device upgrade, lead infection, or ICD dysfunction) as well as the length of time that the leads have been in place. While subclavian vein injuries during explantation can often be repaired with endovascular approaches, more proximal injuries, most commonly to the SVC and less commonly to the RA or RV require cardiac surgical intervention and carry a 36–50% risk of mortality [2, 3].

It is imperative to quickly recognize when a perforation has occurred, so that prompt and directed action can be taken. In the unstable patient undergoing PPM/ICD explant, tamponade physiology should quickly be investigated using a combination of hemodynamic parameters and TEE. The latter will show brisk accumulation of pericardial fluid with collapse of the RA and then ventricle and consequent bowing of the interventricular septum into the left ventricle. This will manifest with increased central venous filling pressures and decreased cardiac output. The patient will thus suffer from quick hemodynamic collapse with equalization of the systolic and diastolic blood pressures and tachycardia progressing to PEA arrest [4].

Prompt surgical action is necessary when tamponade physiology is recognized. Tamponade of SVC lacerations using a compliant endovascular balloon was recently demonstrated to be safe and efficacious in patients with an isolated SVC laceration caused by ICD explanation [3]. However, this method requires definitive localization of the perforation to the SVC, which may not be possible in an actively decompensating patient. Percutaneous drainage of the effusion is tempting as the least invasive option but does not allow for surgical closure of the perforation and will lead to exsanguination and/or ongoing tamponade physiology in the likely event that there is ongoing bleeding and/or inadequate drainage of the large volume partially clotted bloody effusion. In the emergent setting, a sternotomy is considered the primary surgical approach, but subxyphoid pericardial window is a reasonable alternative in some circumstances, particularly when RV perforation is suspected. A subxyphoid pericardial window can be performed quickly and effectively with minimal equipment (scalpel and scissors) to relieve the tamponade and temporize the patient while the OR team prepares the field for an emergent sternotomy and the cardiac perfusion team prepares for CPB. In addition, an RV perforation can sometimes be repaired via the subxyphoid approach, particularly in patients with a small heart. In patients with ongoing bleeding and hemodynamic instability with no identifiable perforation via the subxyphoid approach, injury to the RA and/or SVC should be suspected, and an emergent sternotomy should be performed. The need for CPB after sternotomy is dictated by the extent and location of the injury. Simple perforations on the RV, or the anterior surface of the RA or SVC, are amenable to repair with pledgeted sutures without CPB, whereas complex lacerations that are difficult to visualize and repair quickly, especially in the hemodynamically unstable patient, should be repaired on CPB immediately after systemic heparinization. Aortic cannulation can be performed quickly without a purse string cannulation suture and the patient can be placed on bypass using the Poole suction as a means of venous return. Large lacerations or extension to the posterior surface of the SVC or RA may require separate cannulation of both the SVC and IVC to allow for mobilization of the heart and exclusion of the perforation so that it can be repaired in a bloodless field with the heart mobilized to the left. An option for emergent SVC cannulation that should be kept in mind is passing a 6.5 cuffed endotracheal tube via the right atrial appendage. Inflation of the cuff controls hemorrhage while the lumen is connected to the venous return.

These types of injuries should be repaired with a patch reconstruction to prevent narrowing of the SVC and the subsequent development of SVC syndrome. Adequacy of the patch repair can be confirmed via TEE to ensure there is no significant pressure gradient across the repair. Extra care and attention now will prevent chronic problems in the future, especially if new transvenous leads will be required. The innominate vein should also be inspected, as it is a possible albeit uncommon site for injury and can be repaired or ligated, if necessary.

References

1. Hsu JC, Varosy PD, Bao H, Dewland TA, Curtis JP, Marcus GM. Cardiac perforation from implantable cardioverter-defibrillator lead placement: insights from the national cardiovascular data registry. Circ Cardiovasc Qual Outc. 2013;6(5):582–90.
2. Brunner MP, Cronin EM, Wazni O, Baranowski B, Saliba WI, Sabik JF, et al. Outcomes of patients requiring emergent surgical or endovascular intervention for catastrophic complications during transvenous lead extraction. Heart Rhythm. 2014;11(3):419–25.
3. Azarrafiy R, Tsang DC, Boyle TA, Wilkoff BL, Carrillo RG. Compliant endovascular balloon reduces the lethality of superior vena cava tears during transvenous lead extractions. Heart Rhythm. 2017;14(9):1400–4.
4. Appleton C, Gillam L, Koulogiannis K. Cardiac Tamponade. Cardiol Clin. 2017;35(4):525–37.

Chapter 29
Tube Thoracostomy for Hemothorax

Lynze R. Franko, Kenneth T. Shelton, and Arminder Jassar

Problem

A frail 75-year-old man with a past medical history of atrial fibrillation on apixaban and COPD on home oxygen presents to the ED via ambulance with chest pain and shortness of breath after a fall. On chest X-ray he has a moderately sized hemopneumothorax associated with several left-sided rib fractures. You decide to help the intern place a 14-Fr chest tube utilizing the Seldinger technique. After all, seniors teaching juniors is what it's all about. The insertion location of the tube is selected based on its predicted placement at the 5th intercostal space. While placing the chest tube, a needle and syringe are utilized and blood is aspirated, not unexpected given the hemothorax. The tube slides in without difficulty and you cannot help but smile to yourself.

Just your third month as a CT fellow and you have mastered teaching this skill!

You expected the liter of blood that drained immediately, but not the drop in blood pressure to the 90s. Shouldn't he improve with drainage of the effusion? You are expecting significant bleeding from the patient's apixaban use, but your sense of confidence turns to fear as the color of the blood turns from dark to bright red! You clamp the tube, call for more blood, and head to the CT scanner. The tip of the chest tube is in the left ventricle. No wonder he was hypotensive!

What are you going to do now?

L. R. Franko · A. Jassar (✉)
Department of Surgery, Massachusetts General Hospital, Boston, MA, USA
e-mail: ajassar@mgh.harvard.edu

L. R. Franko
e-mail: Lfranko@mgh.harvard.edu

K. T. Shelton
Department of Anesthesia, Massachusetts General Hospital, Boston, MA, USA
e-mail: kshelton@mgh.harvard.edu

© The Author(s), under exclusive license to Springer Nature Switzerland AG 2022   117
T. M. Sundt et al. (eds.), *Near Misses in Cardiac Surgery*,
https://doi.org/10.1007/978-3-030-92750-9_29

Solution

You suspect this has occurred because the patient's cardiomegaly was underappreciated given the hemothorax. Thankful that you did not elect to place a large bore tube, you call ahead to the OR and then instruct your team to keep the chest tube clamped and in place; removing the tube would likely lead to immediate death from exsanguination. Your hope is that the tube is partially occluding the hole within the left ventricle although it has not escaped your attention that there are side holes in the tube. Time is of the essence. Fortunately, an OR is available, and a crack cardiac anesthesia team has just finished a case.

The patient is rapidly induced, prepped, and draped. You perform a median sternotomy to find a tense pericardium as the attending surgeon arrives from home. It is your complication and your responsibility to fix it, so she steps up to the left side of the table. After clearing blood clots from around the heart, you consider trying to control the site without resorting to cardiopulmonary bypass given the patient's anticoagulation status. It is remarkable how much one can elevate the heart from the pericardial space if the right-sided pericardium is not suspended but rather is permitted to fall, a lesson learned from the off-pump experience. One may even choose to open the right pleural space to prevent compression of the right atrium. But given the patient's significant cardiomegaly you are concerned about turning a controlled situation into uncontrollable bleeding with hypotension if you displace the heart and dislodge the chest tube.

After commencing bypass, you gently lift the apex of the heart with stay sutures, elevating the left pericardium. Luckily, the catheter insertion site into the ventricle is a good distance from the left anterior descending artery. You then remove the catheter, and taking care to avoid the coronary arteries, you repair the ventricular injury with a large felt pledgeted 4.0 prolene on a small half circular (SH) needle, remembering that it is a greater sin to tie this suture too tight than too loose. You cannot afford to turn this puncture into a gaping tear. Better to put in a second stitch than to overdo the first. The patient weans from bypass, and thankfully recovers uneventfully, neurologically intact albeit a bit worse for the wear.

Discussion

Placing a chest tube is not a benign procedure. The reported rate of significant complications of chest tube placement is between 5 and 10% [1, 2]. Some of the most frequent complications during placement include malposition of the tube and technical complications [1, 2]. If placed in a cavity with significant pleural adhesions there may be significant–even torrential–intrapleural hemorrhage. Placement too low risks injury to the liver or spleen, particularly in patients with an elevated diaphragm due to phrenic palsy or obesity [1–3]. Phrenic nerve injury can occur as well as re-expansion edema if the lung has been compressed for an extended period of time. Ultrasound guidance has been shown to reduce the rate of complications and is now commonplace in clinical practice if time permits.[1] In particular, image guidance is recommended in high risk populations, [1–3] such as those patients with previous intrathoracic procedures, pleurodesis, cardiomegaly, ascites, and diaphragmatic muscle dysfunction unless emergency decompression is needed [2, 4]. A clear understanding of the anatomical landmarks is critical for chest tube placement within the triangle of safety [2, 4].

In the case above, there was evidence of left ventricular perforation during pigtail chest tube insertion. When this situation occurs, it is also important to use transesophageal echocardiography (TEE) to carefully assess valve function for damage as this may also require repair [3]. Given that median sternotomy allows for cardiopulmonary bypass and more effective resolution of any remaining pericardial blood, this approach is recommended although emergent left thoracotomy would have been appropriate if the repair had to be attempted in the ED. The decision to repair on cardiopulmonary bypass depends on the location of the perforation, ability to obtain visualization, and hemodynamic stability with manipulation of the heart. Cardiac arrest on CPB may not be required if hemodynamic stability obtained with CPB allows for manipulation of the heart [3]. Of note, if not repaired on CPB, placing the suture prior to removing the catheter may allow for lower blood loss and more precisely placed stitches [3]. Temporary rapid ventricular pacing may also assist in allowing for stitch accuracy when not utilizing CPB [3].

References

1. Mao M, et al. Complications of chest tubes: a focused clinical synopsis. Curr Opin Pulm Med. 2015;21(4):376–86.
2. Filosso PL, et al. Errors and Complications in Chest Tube Placement. Thorac Surg Clin. 2017;27(1):57–67.
3. Varghese S, et al. Surgical Management of Iatrogenic Left Ventricle Perforation by Chest Tube Insertion. Ann Thorac Surg. 2019;108(6):e405–7.
4. Shin-Kim J, et al. Left ventricular perforation with catheter decompression. Am J Emerg Med. 2019;37(2):377.e5-377.e6.

Chapter 30
Pulmonary Hypertension

Corey Spiro and Michael G. Fitzsimons

Problem

You've just finished your fourth cup of coffee for the morning, and you're bursting with energy as you stride confidently into the operating room. Your patient is a 48-year-old woman scheduled for mitral valve repair. She lives in a cabin in the backwoods of Maine and hasn't seen a doctor for decades since she reports having "no medical problems whatsoever" until last week, that is, when she presented to the emergency department with acute shortness of breath. Her chest X-ray revealed moderate pulmonary edema with small pleural effusions, and her NT-pro-BNP was elevated to 4000 pg/mL. Transthoracic echocardiogram showed severe mitral regurgitation, with a focal prolapse of the P2 scallop. Her left ventricular end diastolic diameter was 6.8 cm, indicating this was not entirely new; the left ventricular ejection fraction was 65%. The right ventricle was also moderately dilated with systolic function at the lower limits of normal and moderate tricuspid regurgitation. Regadenoson-MIBI stress test was negative for ischemia. She was admitted to the hospital and diuresed aggressively with intravenous furosemide for several days. As of this morning her chest X-ray is clear, and you're feeling good that she's optimized for surgery (although you notice she appears quite winded after moving herself over onto the operating room table).

Figuring you have time for a fifth cup of coffee while the patient is being induced and lines are placed, you sidle towards the lounge. But moments later, you are

C. Spiro
Department of Anesthesia, Critical Care, and Pain Medicine, Massachusetts General Hospital, Boston, MA, USA

M. G. Fitzsimons (✉)
Division of Cardiac Anesthesia, Department of Anesthesia, Critical Care, and Pain Medicine, Harvard Medical School, Massachusetts General Hospital, Boston, MA, USA
e-mail: MFITZSIMONS@mgh.harvard.edu

© The Author(s), under exclusive license to Springer Nature Switzerland AG 2022
T. M. Sundt et al. (eds.), *Near Misses in Cardiac Surgery*,
https://doi.org/10.1007/978-3-030-92750-9_30

called back to the operating room by your anesthesia colleague, who has just placed a pulmonary artery catheter. The initial hemodynamics are as follows: systemic BP 117/58 mmHg, CVP 20 mmHg, RV 98/18 mmHg, PA 97/42 mmHg, and PCWP of 17 mmHg. The pulmonary vascular resistance is 4 Woods units. The cardiac index by thermodilution is 1.9 L/min/m^2. Given the degree of tricuspid regurgitation, you request that central venous and arterial blood gasses be checked to calculate a Fick cardiac output; the Fick measurement correlates perfectly with the thermodilution value. The anesthesiologist attempts to lower the pulmonary arterial pressures by deepening the anesthetic, titrating PEEP to optimize pulmonary compliance, stopping all alpha-agonists, and hyperventilating the patient with 100% FiO$_2$. Unfortunately, these measures do not lower the PA pressures substantially.

What to do? You are at a fork in the road: proceed with surgery or admit to the ICU?

Solution

You strongly suspect the high pulmonary pressures are a result of the severe mitral regurgitation. Even so, the elevated pulmonary vascular resistance (coupled with your suspicion the disease process has been long-standing) makes you fairly concerned the patient has mixed pre- and post-capillary pulmonary hypertension. Before proceeding with the surgery, you decide to challenge the patient with a pulmonary vasodilator to see whether the high PVR is fixed or reversible. At your request, the anesthesiologist administers a continuous nebulized infusion of inhaled epoprostenol; after several minutes, the PA pressures have decreased to 68/40 and the cardiac index has improved to 2.1 L/min/m^2. Feeling confident the pulmonary vascular remodeling is at least partly reversible; you elect to go ahead with the case.

The mitral repair proceeds uneventfully. You briefly consider placing a tricuspid annuloplasty ring as well; however, you decide against it given your concern that increasing the effective afterload on the right ventricle (not to mention extending the length of the bypass run) could precipitate right ventricular failure in the face of elevated pulmonary vascular pressures.

As you rewarm, you close the left atrium and de-air the heart. Once the aortic cross clamp is removed, you discuss with the anesthesiologist how to support the right ventricle during separation from cardiopulmonary bypass. You agree to resume inhaled epoprostenol in addition to starting infusions of epinephrine and milrinone. The milrinone results in a modest drop in blood pressure which you attribute to a decrease in systemic vascular resistance. You suggest the anesthesiologist begin an infusion of vasopressin as well, with the thought this might counteract the decrease in SVR with minimal effects on pulmonary vascular resistance. Once these drugs are running and the patient is warm, you direct the perfusionist to slowly separate from cardiopulmonary bypass, closely watching the pulmonary artery pressures and central venous pressure as you do so.

Bi-ventricular function is unchanged from before, although the tricuspid regurgitation now appears to be more solidly in the moderate range. However, the pulmonary artery pressure remains elevated at 64/38 mmHg which is somewhat concerning. Protamine is administered very slowly as you decannulate, and fortunately, the hemodynamics remain unchanged. After obtaining hemostasis and closing the chest, the patient is transported to the intensive care unit in stable condition.

The patient is extubated later that afternoon but remains in the intensive care unit for the next several days while the epinephrine, milrinone, epoprostenol, and vasopressin are weaned. You diurese the patient with furosemide, and on postoperative day two a transthoracic echocardiogram shows that the tricuspid regurgitation is now mild; however, the pulmonary artery pressures remain elevated. You consult with a pulmonary hypertension specialist, who recommends starting the patient on oral sildenafil. The patient is discharged on this regimen, and when you see her in your office several weeks later, she reports that her functional status has improved markedly.

Discussion

Normal mean pulmonary artery pressure is 14 mmHg $\pm$ 3. Pulmonary hypertension, defined as a mean pulmonary artery pressure >25 mmHg, is associated with increased morbidity and mortality in cardiac surgical patients. The World Health Organization categorizes pulmonary hypertension into five groups, based on etiology: Group 1 includes patients with elevated pulmonary vascular resistance because of idiopathic disease. Group 2 includes patients with left heart disease, which may reflect LV dysfunction and/or valvular disease. Group 3 includes patients with pulmonary hypertension because of lung disease or chronic hypoxemia. Group 4 represents chronic thromboembolic pulmonary hypertension. Group 5 includes patients with unclear or multifactorial mechanisms.

Alternatively, pulmonary hypertension can be classified as pre-capillary (indicating the presence of increased pulmonary vascular resistance), post-capillary (with normal PVR but elevated pulmonary venous pressures), or mixed. The presence of long-standing post-capillary pulmonary hypertension, as in this scenario, may result in remodeling of the pulmonary vasculature with medial hypertrophy leading to mixed pre- and post-capillary disease, with fixed elevations of pulmonary vascular resistance. Delineation between pre- versus post-capillary disease requires calculation of the pulmonary vascular resistance. Measuring the trans-pulmonary gradient (defined as the difference between mean PA pressure and PCWP) can also be helpful, with a trans-pulmonary gradient >12 mmHg suggesting pulmonary hypertension "out of proportion" to pulmonary venous back-pressures alone.

Making the distinction between pre- and post-capillary hypertension is critical since the therapeutic approach will depend on the underlying mechanism. Patients with post-capillary pulmonary hypertension require therapy for their underlying ventricular failure: diuretics, revascularization, and correction of aortic or mitral valvular disease will decrease pulmonary venous pressures. For patients with pure post-capillary pulmonary hypertension because of mitral valvular disease, the pulmonary pressures would be expected to normalize after mitral valve surgery. On the other hand, patients with pre-capillary pulmonary hypertension will benefit from pulmonary vasodilators. Pulmonary vasodilators commonly used in the peri-operative period include inhaled guanylate cyclase activators such as nitric oxide, inhaled prostaglandins such as epoprostanol, and intravenous phosphodi-esterase inhibitors such as milrinone. A variety of oral agents are also available including endothelin receptor antagonists, guanylate cyclase stimulators, and phosphodiesterase inhibitors.

When pre-capillary pulmonary hypertension is suspected, as was the case for this patient, it may be prudent to employ a pulmonary vasodilator challenge before proceeding with the planned surgery. Knowing whether the elevated PVR is fixed, fully reversible, or partly reversible with pulmonary vasodilators can help inform the decision whether to proceed with the surgery as well as stratify the risk of right heart failure and the difficulty of separating from cardiopulmonary bypass.

Bibliography

1. Farber HW, Loscalzo J. Pulmonary arterial hypertension. N Engl J Med. 2004;351 (16):1655–65.
2. Konstam MA, Kiernan MS, Bernstein D, Bozkurt B, Jacob M, Kapur NK, Kociol RD, Lewis EF, Mehra MR, Pagani FD, Raval AN, Ward C, American Heart Association Council on Clinical Cardiology; Council on Cardiovascular Disease in the Young; and Council on Cardiovascular Surgery and Anesthesia. Evaluation and management of right-sided heart failure: a scientific statement from the American Heart Association. Circulation. 2018;137(20): e578–22.
3. Patel H, Desai M, Tuzcu EM, Griffin B, Kapadia S. Pulmonary hypertension in mitral regurgitation. J Am Heart Assoc. 2014;3(4):e000748.
4. Sarkar MS, Desai PM. Pulmonary hypertension and cardiac anesthesia: anesthesiologist's perspective. Ann Card Anaesth. 2018;21(2):116–22.
5. Zamanian RT, Kudelko KT, Sung YK, Perez VJ, Liu J, Spiekerkoetter E. Current clinical management of pulmonary arterial hypertension. Circ Res. 2014;115(1):131–47.

Chapter 31
Malfunction of an Intra-aortic Balloon

Thoralf M. Sundt and Myles E. Lee

Problem

You are on call today for the service and have just received news of a patient who has been transferred from another hospital with severe three-vessel disease and an intra-aortic balloon pump (IABP) in place. It is a Friday afternoon, and you can foresee your weekend plans being disrupted. You wonder whether the balloon pump was really necessary clinically or if it was more a manifestation of the anxiety of the catheterization team facing a weekend (somehow it seems the incidence of balloon pump insertion goes up as the week wears on). One of your mentors was a great enthusiast for balloons, but you have seen too many cold legs to share his enthusiasm. Besides, once a balloon pump is in place, patients are confined to lying supine in bed with fairly uncomfortable accommodations. But you give yourself a good talking to and remind yourself that everyone is doing their best for the patient. Time to suppress the cynicism and head to the CCU.

On arrival, the 72 year old patient is pain-free, and with nothing but a positive stress test performed more out of patient anxiety than anything else. Cardiac catheterization did indeed demonstrate a significant left main lesion with moderate associated right coronary disease. When you look at the films you realize the referring physician was likely exercising good judgment and breathe a sigh of relief that you made no snide comments on arriving in the unit. The patient is otherwise healthy apart from well-controlled diabetes. You weigh the time it will take you to do a 3-vessel bypass on a Saturday against the discomfort he will experience waiting for your Monday slot. After a brief conversation with the patient, you consent him for surgery in the morning and head home.

T. M. Sundt (✉)
Division of Cardiac Surgery, Massachusetts General Hospital, Boston, MA, USA
e-mail: Tsundt@mgh.harvard.edu

M. E. Lee
Cardiothoracic Surgery, Centinela Hospital Medical Center, Inglewood, CA, USA

© The Author(s), under exclusive license to Springer Nature Switzerland AG 2022   125
T. M. Sundt et al. (eds.), *Near Misses in Cardiac Surgery*,
https://doi.org/10.1007/978-3-030-92750-9_31

At 4:00 A.M. the phone rings. The ICU team has been struggling with the balloon pump for about an hour. They saw some blood in the helium line and called the intensivist who in turn called the interventional cardiologist on call for the evening. After some back-and-forth they identified a cardiology fellow to exchange the balloon pump, but it will not withdraw. Not only is it stuck in the sheath, but the patient's leg is cold. The intensivist is agitated and frustrated. They suggest to the fellow that this is the kind of problem that requires a strong back and weak mind, and the cardiology fellow seems like just the man for the job. As tensions escalate the nurses grow concerned and now they have you on the phone. They want your advice on the best way to deal with the problem.

Solution

You thank the nurse for the call and request to speak with the intensivist. Recognizing that his anxiety springs from concern for the patient, you reassure them that given the patient's anatomy you believe he will tolerate withdrawal of balloon pump support just fine. You explain that your greatest concern now is the patient's extremity ischemia. You ask the team to book an operating room with fluoroscopy, where you will be able to explore the femoral artery and external iliac under ideal circumstances. Once you identify the exact location of the balloon pump by flouro you will obtain proximal and distal control and remove the balloon directly. Recognizing that breakfast time is just around the corner, you tell the OR team to just plan on proceeding with coronary bypass once the balloon is out. You chalk it up to an early start on the weekend giving you an opportunity to cook pancakes for the kids after all. You may even get a chance to watch Brady win yet another football game.

Discussion

The incidence of significant complications of intra-aortic balloon pumps will of course depend upon your definition of significance, but they are certainly not uncommon. A remarkably simple but effective technology that was introduced in the 1960s, it has undoubtedly saved many lives; but equally it has threatened many limbs. Ischemic complications can occur particularly in patients with small or atherosclerotic femoral vessels. For this reason, one must be extraordinarily attentive to distal perfusion after inserting a balloon pump. In some instances, one may choose to insert the balloon without a sheath to minimize luminal compromise of the femoral artery. Other complications include retroperitoneal bleeding at the time of withdrawal due to a high puncture as well as end organ ischemia secondary to cholesterol embolization if the descending thoracic aorta is heavily diseased.

In this instance, however, the complication is a consequence of structural failure of the balloon itself. Balloon rupture is uncommon, but when it does occur, it must be recognized promptly and dealt with expeditiously. This problem can be recognized by the presence of blood in the helium channel for balloon inflation or by drive line helium leak or high pressure alarms. If recognized quickly, a guidewire can be passed through the central lumen, the ruptured balloon removed, and a new balloon passed over the wire. Infusion of streptokinase with a heparinized saline flush into the gas line has also been described if diagnosis is made promptly. If recognized more than 60 min after rupture, however, the blood in the lumen will harden and obstruct gas flow, preventing complete decompression of the balloon and making its removal problematic. Once this is the case, the solution is surgical cutdown, ideally in the operating room if the patient is sufficiently stable. A hard pull will certainly not be enough to pass the balloon through the sheath and depending on the state of the balloon may result in iliac or femoral vessel rupture or even avulsion, a catastrophic event.

Lagniappe

Problem

You have just finished the last steri-strip on your morning case when the overhead page comes through "anesthesia STAT room 47." You know what that means. They are not just calling for anesthesia. They are calling for cardiac anesthesia. And the reason they are calling is serious trouble. You leave the resident to transport the patient to the intensive care unit while you call the family and dictate the case. Just after you have hung up with the spouse, the anesthesia tech finds you at your workstation and asks if you can come to 47. You arrive to find CPR ongoing. The patient is 69 years old and undergoing a radical prostatectomy. The first thought to come to your mind is intraoperative pulmonary embolism, but there is no echo and, no two ways about it, the patient is in profound shock. The cardiothoracic chief resident is already on the scene having just inserted an intra-aortic balloon pump percutaneously but there is no augmentation apparent on the arterial line when they hold CPR. How dilated is this guy?

Solution

You suspect your eager resident has mistakenly cannulated the femoral vein rather than the femoral artery, an easy mistake to make with ongoing CPR since neither pulsatility nor, necessarily, the color of the blood is definitive proof the target has been cannulated. The cardiac anesthesia team has rolled an echo probe into the room and as they introduce it you ask them to take a quick look for the balloon in the right atrium. They confirm your suspicion. You then percutaneously cannulate the artery just 1 cm laterally and they confirm a wire in the descending thoracic aorta. With a balloon pump in place, life-sustaining blood pressure can be maintained. With no evidence of pulmonary embolism, a presumptive diagnosis of acute coronary syndrome is made, and the patient is whisked off to the cardiac catheterization lab.

Discussion

Under ideal circumstances an intra-aortic balloon pump is placed under echocardiographic guidance or fluoroscopy to allow you to confirm the vessel into which the balloon is placed as well as its actual location immediately distal to the left subclavian artery. After cannulating the common femoral artery, a wire is passed and its location in the descending thoracic aorta confirmed before passing dilators and finally the balloon. Of all the steps, cannulating the common femoral artery must not be trivialized. As in this case, distinguishing between the artery and vein can be problematic in the setting of cardiac arrest or low cardiac output state with high central venous pressure where the venous return may appear brisk and pulsatile. The location of the puncture must be correct as well, neither too high nor too low. If too low and in the superficial femoral artery, it may occlude the vessel, while if too high it may lead to life-threatening retroperitoneal hemorrhage. For this reason, it is commonplace today to use ultrasound imaging to identify the target vessel whenever time and available technology permit.

Bibliogrpahy

1. Mizrahi I, Bose S, Leibowitz A. Management of intra-aortic balloon rupture and entrapment. Case Rep J Cardiothorac Vasc Anesth. 2019;33(7):1983–7. https://doi.org/10.1053/j.jvca.2018.08.023. Epub 2018 Aug 17. PMID: 30243865 DOI: https://doi.org/10.1053/j.jvca.2018.08.023.
2. Fitzmaurice GJ, Collins A, Parissis H. Management of intra-aortic balloon pump entrapment: a case report and review of the literature. Tex Heart Inst J. 2012;39(5):621–6. PMID: 2310975.
3. Meharwal ZS, Trehan N. Vascular complications of intra-aortic balloon insertion in patients undergoing coronary reavscularization: analysis of 911 cases. Eur J Cardiothorac Surg. 2002;21:741–7. PMID: 11932177. https://doi.org/10.1016/s1010-7940(02)00034-9.

Chapter 32
Symptomatic Aortic Stenosis

Thoralf Sundt

Problem

You have just been referred a 63-year-old woman with symptomatic aortic stenosis for consideration of aortic valve replacement. Her cardiologic evaluation, complete with cardiac catheterization, was performed at an outside hospital and demonstrates no significant coronary artery disease. You are meeting her for the first time by video teleconference which has become your go-to strategy for patients referred from a distance. It sure is convenient, but it denies you the ability to conduct a complete physical exam. In this day and age, with advanced cardiac imaging, who needs a physical exam anyway? At least that was your thinking until you reviewed her echocardiogram. Her aortic valve leaflets are thickened and certainly do not open normally, but you have seen much worse. There is virtually no calcium on the leaflets. Her ventricular function is normal if not hyperdynamic and her mean gradient is 43 mmHg. But something is not adding up and the stakes are high. Not only are you concerned about subjecting a patient needlessly to the low albeit real risks associated with open heart surgery, but her annulus also looks small. Will you be able to insert a large enough prosthesis to make her feel better?

Solution

Taking advantage of the Heart Team Valve Conference that was established when you participated in the transcatheter valve trials, you present the patient to the group to get some other perspectives. Of course, all are wishing they had the opportunity to examine her, but for this case the team will need to develop a hypothesis based

T. Sundt (✉)
Division of Cardiac Surgery, Massachusetts General Hospital, Boston, MA, USA
e-mail: tsundt@mgh.harvard.edu

© The Author(s), under exclusive license to Springer Nature Switzerland AG 2022   129
T. M. Sundt et al. (eds.), *Near Misses in Cardiac Surgery*,
https://doi.org/10.1007/978-3-030-92750-9_32

on the limited data at its disposal. Fortunately, one of the senior cardiologists is present. A fan of murder mysteries, this is right up her alley. After a bit of discussion, she leans back in her chair and inquires if the patient is on dialysis. "Yes, as a matter of fact. She became symptomatic shortly after her arteriovenous fistula matured. Why do you ask?" She responds that she has previously seen a patient on dialysis found to have a pelvic AV fistula, the combination of which led to a high output state and symptomatic pseudoaortic stenosis. In that case the diagnosis was not made until after the valve replacement. She will not be fooled again. Abdominal and pelvic CTA confirms the diagnosis of a pelvic AV fistula which is embolized with resolution of the patient's symptoms. You have been saved, once again, by the Heart Team.

Discussion

It is important to remember that transvalvular gradients depend not only on the orifice but also on flow through that orifice. Of course, much more commonly, this presents itself as the converse issue, where significant aortic stenosis may be difficult to diagnose because of low flow. When low flow aortic stenosis is suspected, a dobutamine echo can be obtained to look for an increase in gradient. In this case, however, the opposite is true. Without addressing the underlying source of the high flow state, aortic valve replacement is worse than useless, it is potentially harmful given the requisite outflow tract obstruction caused by the valve housing mechanism. Additionally, in a patient on dialysis the risk of subsequent prosthetic endocarditis is very real. In a case like this one, it is simple enough to reassess the gradient while compressing the dialysis fistula. In other cases, the fistula may not be apparent and diagnosis may be difficult. The best next step is cardiac heart catheterization. While Cath Lab hemodynamics are ever more rarely used and cardiologists capable of performing sophisticated hemodynamic assessments a vanishing breed, the key to making this diagnosis would have been right heart catheterization with cardiac output. Her extraordinarily high cardiac output would have tipped one off to the diagnosis, initiating a search for the offending fistula.

Bibliography

1. Ennezat PV, Maréchaux S, Pibarot P. From excessive high-flow, high-gradient to paradoxical low-flow, low-gradient aortic valve stenosis: hemodialysis arteriovenous fistula model. Cardiology. 2010;116(1):70–2. https://doi.org/10.1159/000314938. Epub 2010 May 26 PMID: 205020132.
2. Alkhouli M, Alasfar S, Samuels LA. Valvular heart disease and dialysis access: a case of cardiac decompensation after fistula creation. J Vasc Access. 2013;14(1):96. https://doi.org/10.5301/jva.5000094. Epub 2012 Jul 26. PMID: 22865537.

Chapter 33
Pulmonary Embolism

Thoralf M. Sundt

Problem

Members of the divisions of cardiac surgery, cardiology and pulmonary medicine have just established a pulmonary embolism response team (PERT) whereby anyone in the hospital can request a multidisciplinary video teleconference to discuss management of a patient with PE. You are on call when a page goes out for presentation of a 56 year-old man who fell from a construction site 10 days ago, breaking his femur and sustaining a mild concussion. The trauma orthopedists made quick work of it, discharging the patient after only 4 days in hospital. He returns now to the emergency room with acute onset of shortness of breath—a classic history for pulmonary embolism. Emergency department physicians have obtained a CT scan demonstrating submassive saddle PE and an echocardiogram demonstrating right ventricular strain. Despite this, the patient looks remarkably well on a 2 L nasal cannula at rest and requires no inotropic support. The team wants your input. Heparin, lysis, percutaneous extraction, surgery? What would you recommend?

Solution

Appreciative that the team still regards surgery as an option for the treatment of acute pulmonary embolism, you must admit, with the patient looking so well clinically, it is tough to argue for a sternotomy. His history of head injury gives you pause as well, just as it inspires reluctance to pursue lytic therapy among your medical colleagues. The alternative of low-dose catheter-directed lytic therapy is

T. M. Sundt (✉)
Division of Cardiac Surgery, Massachusetts General Hospital, Boston, MA, USA
e-mail: Tsundt@mgh.harvard.edu

© The Author(s), under exclusive license to Springer Nature Switzerland AG 2022
T. M. Sundt et al. (eds.), *Near Misses in Cardiac Surgery*,
https://doi.org/10.1007/978-3-030-92750-9_33

entertained but the risk still seems uncertain given his apparent clinical stability. Knowing that everything is just fine until it is not, you advocate for anticipatory placement of 7 Fr cannulae in the right common femoral artery and vein after ultrasound demonstrates no local thrombus and admission to the Medical ICU on heparin just in case emergent cannulation for ECMO is required. You have seen how quickly patients can decompensate. Much to your relief, 48 h later the patient's echocardiogram demonstrates improvement in RV function, and after placement of an inferior vena cava filter, he is discharged to the floor.

Discussion

The management of pulmonary embolism in the current era is multidisciplinary. For many years, PE was treated as a complacently accepted yet potentially fatal complication of hospitalization, immobilization, or hypo/hypercoagulable states, but the explosion of percutaneous technologies addressing a variety of cardiovascular diseases has impacted this condition as well. With the advent of percutaneous devices to aspirate thrombus as well as endovascular ultrasound devices intended to accelerate clot dissolution with low-dose lytics, interest in the condition has piqued among physicians who now have an ever broadening number of options.

There has also been a resurgence in interest in the surgical treatment of this condition, the very inspiration for the life's work of John and Mary Gibbon, who developed the machine that evolved directly into our currently used cardiopulmonary bypass pumps. When surgical embolectomy is undertaken, care must be exercised to clear both right and left pulmonary arteries. While the left can be easily accessed centrally, adequate exposure of the right pulmonary artery requires retraction of the aorta away from the superior vena cava permitting a right pulmonary arteriotomy immediately proximal to its arborization. Trying to reach around the aorta from an arteriotomy in the main pulmonary artery will not clear the right lung. Indeed, inadequate extraction of clot may in part have contributed to the poor results that led to an unfounded loss of enthusiasm for surgical embolectomy.

Recognizing the complexity of decision-making given this plethora of complementary approaches, the concept of a pulmonary embolism response team (PERT) has evolved in many institutions. Once a patient with pulmonary embolism is identified, the team is notified, and an ad hoc video teleconference discussion is organized with presentation of history, exam, and imaging studies. This concept has been widely embraced and affords a pathway to achieve greater consensus around the optimal management of a condition which remains remarkably controversial. In this case, right ventricular strain encouraged consideration of more aggressive therapy. Although frightening to look at, the amount of central thrombus itself is not an indication for intervention, and with experience one can appreciate dramatic variation in the amount of physical obstruction that does or does not lead to hemodynamic shock. This is no doubt due to the significant component of vasoconstrictive physiology that accompanies acute pulmonary embolism. The patient's history of head injury, however, steered the team away from either surgical intervention or lytic therapy. Findings of a patent foramen ovale with embolus in transit or, for that matter, right atrial thrombus absent patent foramen ovale, would push one toward surgical intervention, although in the latter some would advocate for an attempt at percutaneous aspiration.

In this case, admission to the intensive care unit with close observation was the right decision coupled with preparatory cannulation of the femoral artery and vein in case hemodynamic collapse occurred, permitting institution of ECMO support. It is worth noting that, given the significant contribution of pulmonary vasoconstriction to the hemodynamic collapse observed with pulmonary embolism, there is also growing enthusiasm for ECMO support in other settings such as pulmonary embolism if the thrombus appears distal or if the patient has received, but failed, lytic therapy, in which case an open surgical procedure can lead to catastrophic bleeding.

Bibliography

1. Effoe VS, Kumar G, Sachdeva R. Intravascular ultrasound-guided pulmonary artery embolectomy for saddle pulmonary embolism. Catheter Cardiovasc Interv. 2020. https://doi.org/10.1002/ccd.28985. PMID: 32432829.
2. Tan CW, Balla S, Ghanta RK, Sharma AM, Chatterjee S. Contemporary management of acute pulmonary embolism. Semin Thorac Cardiovasc Surg. 2020 Autumn;32(3):396–403. https://doi.org/10.1053/j.semtcvs.2020.04.002. PMID: 32353408 Review.
3. Guliani S, Das Gupta J, Osofsky R, Kraai EP, Mitchell JA, Dettmer TS, Wray TC, Tawil I, Rana MA, Marinaro J. Venoarterial extracorporeal membrane oxygenation is an effective management strategy for massive pulmonary embolism patients. J Vasc Surg Venous Lymphat Disord. 2020:S2213-333X(20)30321-8. https://doi.org/10.1016/j.jvsv.2020.04.033. PMID: 32505687; Melamed R, St Hill CA, Engstrom BI, Tierney DM, Smith CS, Agboto VK, Weise BE, Eckman PM, Skeik N. Effects of a consensus-based pulmonary embolism treatment algorithm and response team on treatment modality choices, outcomes, and complications. Clin Appl Thromb Hemost. 2020;26:1076029620928420. https://doi.org/10.1177/1076029620928420. PMID: 32539524.
4. Stępniewski J, Kopeć G, Musiałek P, Magoń W, Jonas K, Waligóra M, Sobczyk D, Podolec P. Hemodynamic effects of ultrasound-assisted, catheter-directed, very low-dose, short-time duration thrombolysis in acute intermediate-high risk pulmonary embolism (from the EKOS-PL study). Am J Cardiol. 2020:S0002-9149(20)31228-5. https://doi.org/10.1016/j.amjcard.2020.11.004. PMID: 33220318.

Chapter 34
Post-operative Bleeding

Greg A. Leya, Kenneth T. Shelton, and Arminder Jassar

Problem

You were delighted to finish your surgical week with a straightforward CABG ×3 in a slender 72 year-old gentleman with nice targets and a normal ventricle. What was commonplace a decade ago now seems rare! You placed the left internal thoracic artery to the left anterior descending, of course, and passed the right internal thoracic artery through the transverse sinus to a large obtuse marginal. The right coronary was not critically stenosed, so you used a vein rather than a radial artery. You dropped the patient off in the ICU at 5 pm. and still had time for dinner with friends.

As you walk in the front door of your house, you get a call from the ICU. The patient has put out 350 cc of blood from his chest tubes in the first hour. You are concerned but knowing that you were in both pleural spaces you ask yourself whether you adequately evacuated both before closing the chest. Much to your relief, the patient puts out 150 cc in the next hour followed by 100 cc the hour after that. Just as you are finishing dinner, your pager goes off again. The patient has just put out 280 cc for a total of 880 cc since the OR. The nurses tell you they had just finished rolling the patient side to side and that he had coughed a bit. The tubes are patent, and you rationalize that this was just an undrained collection. The next hour's output is 100 cc, followed by 210 cc, and then 70 cc. The patient's cardiac filling pressures by pulmonary artery catheter are low and the cardiac output/index

G. A. Leya · A. Jassar (✉)
Department of Surgery, Massachusetts General Hospital, Boston, MA, USA
e-mail: ajassar@mgh.harvard.edu

G. A. Leya
e-mail: gleya@mgh.harvard.edu

K. T. Shelton
Department of Anesthesia, Massachusetts General Hospital, Boston, MA, USA
e-mail: kshelton@mgh.harvard.edu

© The Author(s), under exclusive license to Springer Nature Switzerland AG 2022   135
T. M. Sundt et al. (eds.), *Near Misses in Cardiac Surgery*,
https://doi.org/10.1007/978-3-030-92750-9_34

is good. There is no evidence of clinical tamponade, but the bleeding is irksome, fluctuating hour to hour.

Without doubt the primary driver of your decision is what you believe is best for the patient. Still you cannot help but consider what this will look like at a mortality and morbidity conference. Another takeback? Aren't you drying the patients up before closing? Are you in that much of a hurry? The division has focused on its quality metrics and takeback for bleeding seems to be the Chief's favorite topic these days. On the other hand, next month she may be focused on blood product utilization. Either way it is pretty clear this straightforward case has become a lesson in humility. What to do?

Solution

Of all the complications you have faced in your young career, postoperative bleeding is simultaneously the most common and the most irksome. After a beautiful operation, to have to go back for hemorrhage is a bitter pill to swallow. The enthusiasm of your colleagues in cardiology for antiplatelet agents and novel anticoagulants seems to only make this worse. But you know better than to look for sympathy there. So, you buck-up and take the patient back to the operating room to find bleeding from the toe of the right internal mammary artery (RIMA) graft to the obtuse marginal branch of the circumflex.

It was a beautiful arterial graft and you certainly do not want to compromise the anastomosis, but re-heparinizing for bypass is equally unappealing so, you ask for the off-pump suction stabilizer system, elevate the heart, and carefully place one perfect simple suture in the toe. Hemostasis! You return the heart to the chest and carefully inspect the rest of the mediastinum. The only thing worse than coming back for bleeding is coming back for bleeding twice! You close the incision and return the patient to the ICU. Now you can get some sleep.

Discussion

The causes of postoperative bleeding may be technical, as in this case, or secondary to coagulopathy. Whereas technical bleeding is more likely to require a return to the OR, coagulopathic bleeding is more appropriately managed in the ICU. While less common in off-pump coronary artery bypass procedures, coagulopathic bleeding can be caused by a plethora of factors, including hypothermia, residual or rebound heparin effects post-cardiopulmonary bypass, hemodilution from the crystalloid prime, or fibrinolysis from bypass circuit contact, among other factors not to mention more common use of novel anticoagulants or NOACS.

Re-operation rates vary from 1 to 5%. Not surprisingly, the incidence of reoperation for bleeding differs significantly among cardiac surgical procedures. Without a doubt, we most often find ourselves re-exploring patients after coronary bypass, but that is because this remains the most common operation that we perform. While aortic valve replacement (AVR) may seem a more straightforward operation than coronary bypass, where there are more opportunities for bleeding from conduit side arms and harvest beds, the incidence of reoperation is twice as high for AVR as it is for CABG according to the Society of Thoracic Surgeons database, possibly secondary to the effects of Heyde syndrome wherein platelet activation by the high velocity jet of aortic stenosis causes acquired von Willebrand's disease.

Regardless, every cardiac surgeon is going to face the challenge of dealing with postoperative bleeding. It is discouraging when the patient looks dry in the operating room but upon arrival in the ICU puts out an enormous volume of blood. In such cases, the decision is simple: return to the operating room. The same is true when there is evidence of tamponade (elevated CVP, rising inotropic and vasopressor requirements). The patient presented in this case poses a more challenging problem, with chest tube output up one hour and down the next. For this reason, it is important to establish a regular decision-making framework and standardized data points to aid your thought process. A routine post-operative CXR and coagulation studies, along with standardized chest tube output thresholds for consideration of takeback, can help in your decision-making. Some surgeons abide by the rule of > 400 cc × 1 h, >300 cc × 2–3 h, or >200 cc × 4 h, whereas others set a hard cutoff of 1000 cc of total output. Of course, such levels depend upon whether the pleural spaces have been opened and if the pleural spaces have been adequately drained at the completion of the operative case, as well as chest tube positioning and changes in patient position. Remember Shumway's rule: air rises and blood finds its lowest level! Without strict bleeding cutoffs, however, you can easily find, having bargained with yourself all night long, an embarrassing amount of chest tube output in the morning. The result may be that the patient requires transfusions that would otherwise not have been needed. Ultimately, however, the decision to go back to the OR factors in many other variables, including the patient's hemodynamic status and the pattern of chest tube drainage.

An appropriate resuscitation strategy is important to consider before returning to the OR. Because coagulopathy begets more coagulopathy, the longer you sit on a patient, the more dire the situation may get. While there is no standardized "safe" hemoglobin cutoff, most surgeons transfuse to a Hg goal of 7.0 in a stable patient. Nonetheless, in a bleeding patient, a higher goal of 8 may be more appropriate to facilitate oxygen transport, especially if the MVO_2 is marginal or there are other signs of ischemia. Important adjuncts include adequately re-warming the patient, treating hypertension, or increasing PEEP for a tamponade effect on bleeding. Based on the PTT, platelet count, INR, and fibrinogen levels, administration of protamine, platelets, FFP, cryoprecipitate, Amicar, or tranexamic acid is also appropriate. PRBC or whole blood transfusions, of course, are not without their known risks. Numerous studies have demonstrated the association between transfusion and increased patient mortality, likely secondary to factors including volume overload and TACO (transfusion-related circulatory overload), inflammatory processes like TRALI (transfusion-related acute lung injury), and immune dysregulation from cytokines. Ultimately, however, for bleeding consistent with a technical complication, there is nothing better than early re-exploration for management, with demonstrable improvements in patient morbidity and mortality compared to delayed takeback.

Even with early re-exploration, it is common to find no particular source of bleeding. And yet exploring the chest, evacuating the blood, and irrigating copiously seems to correct the problem, perhaps by correcting a localized DIC. In this instance you found a specific bleeder. The challenge was to repair the anastomosis without compromising it. This is one instance where the use of off-pump stabilizers has simplified our lives tremendously. If none are available, you may indeed have to re-heparinize and go back on bypass to place that critical stitch.

Learning Objectives

(1) Understand chest tube output and when to re-explore (hemodynamic parameters, tamponade as a clinical diagnosis)
(2) Understand bleeding spaces (pericardial, pleural, abdominal) and diagnosis/management
(3) Bleeding resuscitation and complications of resuscitation (volume overload, TACO/TRALI, immune regulation).

Bibliography

1. Patel K, Adalti S, Runwal S, Singh R, Ananthanrayanan C, Doshi C, Pandya H. Re-exploration after off-pump coronary artery bypass grafting: incidence, risk factors, and impact of timing. J Card Surg. 2020;35(11):3062–9.
2. Biancari F, Kinnunen E-M, Kiviniemi T, Tauriainen T, Anttila V, Airaksinen JKE, Brascia D, Vasques F. Meta-analysis of the sources of bleeding after adult cardiac surgery. J Cardiothorac Vasc Anesth. 2018;32(4):1618–24.
3. Frojd V, Jeppson A. Re-exploration for bleeding and its association with mortality after cardiac surgery. Ann Thorac Surg. 2016;102(1):109–17.
4. Society of Thoracic Surgeons Blood Conversation Guidelines Task Force, Ferraris VA et al. 2011 update to the society of thoracic surgeons and the society of cardiovascular anesthesiologists blood conservation clinical practice guideline. Ann Thorac Surg. 2011;91(3).
5. Spiess BD. Choose one: damned if you do/damned if you don't! Crit Care Med. 2005;33:1871–3.
6. Murphy GJ, Angelini GD. Indications for blood transfusion in cardiac surgery. Ann Thorac Surg. 2006;82:2323–34.
7. Scott BH, Seifert FC, Grimson R. Blood transfusion is associated with increased resource utilisation, morbidity and mortality in cardiac surgery. Ann Card Anaesth. 2008;11:15–9.
8. Reeves BC, Murphy GJ. Increased mortality, morbidity, and cost associated with red blood cell transfusion after cardiac surgery. Curr Opin Anaesthesiol. 2008;21:669–73.

Chapter 35
Intraoperative Extracorporeal Cardiopulmonary Resuscitation

Travis Hull and Masaki Funamoto

Problem

You are delighted to be leaving the hospital early after a light schedule in the OR. It's a perfect autumn day. The sun is warm and there is a cool breeze outside. Just as you are about to leave the hospital early and head off to the country club for a round of golf, you receive a STAT intraoperative extracorporeal cardiopulmonary resuscitation (eCPR) consult to room 41 where a 46 year-old man is undergoing pneumonectomy for locally advanced recurrent lung cancer with right atrial and esophageal invasion. When you arrive in the operating room, the patient is in the left lateral decubitus position with a generous posterior right thoracotomy, having tolerated right pneumonectomy with partial esophageal wall and left atrial cuff resection as well. The bronchial cuff and esophageal wall defect are beautifully buttressed with an omental flap harvested via a right subcostal abdominal incision. All was well until the team begins to close the abdominal incision when the patient suddenly and acutely deteriorates with ST elevations on EKG followed by PEA arrest. What a turn of events after 10 h of surgery with success in sight! When you arrive, the thoracic surgery team is performing chest compressions the best they can despite the decubitus position.

T. Hull
Department of Surgery, Massachusetts General Hospital, Boston, MA, USA
e-mail: Thull1@partners.org

M. Funamoto (✉)
Department of Cardiothoracic Surgery, Methodist Hospital, San Antonio, USA

© The Author(s), under exclusive license to Springer Nature Switzerland AG 2022
T. M. Sundt et al. (eds.), *Near Misses in Cardiac Surgery*,
https://doi.org/10.1007/978-3-030-92750-9_35

Solution

You quickly scrub in and open the pericardium widely so you can perform direct manual cardiac message using a two-handed technique to avoid myocardial injury or RVOT compression. You are able to maintain a perfusing blood pressure with a pulsatile A-line tracing showing a MAP of 60 mm Hg. You ask for cardiac anesthesia to be consulted STAT for intra-operative transesophageal echocardiography (TEE) just as the patient fibrillates. Mechanical support will clearly be required. You ask for heparin to be administered and instruct the senior thoracic surgery fellow to cannulate the femoral vessels for peripheral veno-arterial extracorporeal membrane oxygenation (VA-ECMO). In this way, effective cardiac massage can be maintained without risking an air embolism associated with central ECMO cannulation. A 19 Fr arterial cannula is passed percutaneously over a wire followed by a 23/25 Fr venous drainage cannula over a Super Stiff Amplatz wire in the right femoral vein after TEE confirms the wire to be in the right atrium. With initiation of VA-ECMO, flow is insufficient to maintain MAP > 55 mm Hg. The patient remains in persistent VF despite multiple attempts to defibrillate with internal paddles. Reaching inside the pericardial space, the LV feels full. You know you will not be able to defibrillate a distended ventricle, so you perform manual compression it to empty it out. With this, the patient converts to sinus rhythm at which time flows increase in excess of 4 L per minute. The situation is now under control. You inspect the surgical field and place temporary epicardial A&V pacing leads. Your thoracic colleagues close the large defect in the pericardium with vicryl mesh to prevent cardiac herniation and temporarily close the thoracotomy incision. Your last step is to place a 6 Fr distal Perfusor in the right superficial femoral artery under ultrasound guidance before securing all the cannulas in place. The patient is sent directly to the cardiac catheterization laboratory where two critical right coronary artery stenoses are dilated. After formal chest closure, the ECMO circuit is reconfigured to venoarterial-venous and subsequently to veno-venous for lung-protective ventilation. With recovery of lung function, he is decannulated and, after a prolonged course, the patient is discharged with plans to continue oncologic therapy for his lung cancer.

Discussion

eCPR is an established method of cardiopulmonary resuscitation in patients who suffer cardiac arrest in the inpatient setting, and as such, its use is rapidly growing [1, 2]. eCPR is defined as VA-ECMO offered as the initial means of resuscitation from cardiac arrest in patients who fail to achieve sustained return of spontaneous circulation (ROSC) by conventional CPR [3]. eCPR is distinct from the VA-ECMO support offered to patients suffering from cardiogenic shock due to acute myocardial infarction or myocarditis, RV failure, congenital heart disease, cardiomyopathy, refractory ventricular tachycardia, failure to wean from cardiopulmonary bypass, post-cardiotomy shock, or acute or chronic graft dysfunction after transplantation. The most important determinant of success of eCPR is immediate institution of basic life support (BLS) including CPR such that no-flow time is <5 min. Additionally, institution of eCPR within 20 min of arrest is critical [4, 5].

Broadly speaking, eCPR and VA-ECMO can be instituted as a bridge-to-recovery (depending on the extent of end organ insult, and therefore, survivability after an arrest), to a more durable means of mechanical circulatory support or to transplantation [6]. eCPR is generally reserved for young patients (ideally less than 60) who have suffered a witnessed arrest with an initial rhythm of VF or VT and where BLS is instituted within 5 min but fails to achieve ROSC within 15 min. eCPR is withheld from patients with asystole as their initial rhythm, as well as those who have an unwitnessed arrest, total arrest time > 60 min, severe pre-existing conditions or contraindications to anticoagulation, acute aortic dissection, hemorrhagic or other non-cardiogenic shock, and those who are DNR [6]. The absolute and relative contraindications for eCPR are often difficult to fully assess in the critically ill patient who requires prompt intervention. It should not be offered to patients with no meaningful chance of recovery, which can be difficult to evaluate in the emergent setting, such as the patient in the case above who is young and had immediate institution of conventional CPR but has metastatic lung cancer.

Institution of central ECMO is appealing in patients with an open chest in the operating room and is a good option for those patients already on cardiopulmonary bypass (CPB). However, several factors should be considered when deciding on cannulation for central versus peripheral ECMO in patients not on CPB. In this particular patient, who was sub-optimally positioned for central cannulation and actively dependent on cardiac massage to maintain perfusion, peripheral cannulation was a better choice. While central arterial cannulation can be performed in this patient, central venous cannulation should be avoided due to the disastrous complication of air suction embolism, which is fatal. In addition, the risks of bleeding, transfusion dependence, and need for renal replacement therapy is lower in peripheral compared to central VA-ECMO for eCPR [7].

Cardiac massage through a right thoracotomy is difficult. First, the pericardium must be opened widely since the heart cannot be delivered through it directly such as in the circumstance of a resuscitative anterolateral left thoracotomy. This requires careful attention to avoiding a phrenic nerve injury. A two-handed technique using the flat surface of the hands is optimal to avoid RVOT compression, but a single hand inserted in the inferolateral position to achieve direct compression on the LV is also possible. The efficacy of the chosen massage technique can be monitored based on patient hemodynamics and by assessing the A-line tracing. In addition, given that the pericardiotomy needed to perform cardiac massage via right thoracotomy must be large, it should be closed at the end of the case with a patch reconstruction to prevent cardiac herniation and associated hemodynamic collapse.

An additional important and life-saving consideration in this patient is manual LV venting to break the cycle of ventricular distention and VF/VT storm. This will be marked by inability to achieve forward flow even at low ECMO settings due to suction events from low cardiac output and consequently low venous return. Electrical (defibrillation) and pharmacologic interventions in this scenario will not be successful unless excess wall tension is released manually with LV decompression, which often allows for sinus rhythm to be achieved with a single subsequent application of internal defibrillation. LV venting is particularly important with institution of VA-ECMO, because retrograde blood flow from the arterial cannula increases afterload and can acutely worsen LV distension [8].

References

1. Chen YS, Lin JW, Yu HY, Ko WJ, Jerng JS, Chang WT, et al. Cardiopulmonary resuscitation with assisted extracorporeal life-support versus conventional cardiopulmonary resuscitation in adults with in-hospital cardiac arrest: an observational study and propensity analysis. Lancet. 2008;372(9638):554–61.
2. Shin TG, Choi JH, Jo IJ, Sim MS, Song HG, Jeong YK, et al. Extracorporeal cardiopulmonary resuscitation in patients with inhospital cardiac arrest: a comparison with conventional cardiopulmonary resuscitation. Crit Care Med. 2011;39(1):1–7.
3. Link MS, Berkow LC, Kudenchuk PJ, Halperin HR, Hess EP, Moitra VK, et al. Part 7: Adult advanced cardiovascular life support: 2015 American heart association guidelines update for cardiopulmonary resuscitation and emergency cardiovascular care. Circulation. 2015;132(18 Suppl 2):S444-64.
4. Rajan S, Wissenberg M, Folke F, Hansen SM, Gerds TA, Kragholm K, et al. Association of bystander cardiopulmonary resuscitation and survival according to ambulance response times after out-of-hospital cardiac arrest. Circulation. 2016;134(25):2095–104.
5. Reynolds JC, Frisch A, Rittenberger JC, Callaway CW. Duration of resuscitation efforts and functional outcome after out-of-hospital cardiac arrest: when should we change to novel therapies? Circulation. 2013;128(23):2488–94.
6. Guglin M, Zucker MJ, Bazan VM, Bozkurt B, El Banayosy A, Estep JD, et al. Venoarterial ECMO for adults: JACC scientific expert panel. J Am Coll Cardiol. 2019;73 (6):698–716.
7. Raffa GM, Kowalewski M, Brodie D, Ogino M, Whitman G, Meani P, et al. Meta-analysis of peripheral or central extracorporeal membrane oxygenation in postcardiotomy and non-postcardiotomy shock. Ann Thorac Surg. 2019;107(1):311–21.
8. Annamalai SK, Buiten L, Esposito ML, Paruchuri V, Mullin A, Breton C, et al. Acute hemodynamic effects of intra-aortic balloon counterpulsation pumps in advanced heart failure. J Card Fail. 2017;23(8):606–14.

Chapter 36
Mitral Annular Calcification

Antonia Kreso and Serguei I. Melnitchouk

Problem

A 77-year-old female presented with a history of long-standing moderate mitral stenosis and atrial fibrillation (AF) [1]. Her other medical history was notable for chronic kidney disease and peripheral vascular disease. She has had worsening shortness of breath and dyspnea on exertion. Transthoracic echocardiogram showed progression of the mitral stenosis to severe. Pre-operative workup included transthoracic echocardiogram, showing an ejection fraction of 60%. The mitral valve had a peak gradient of 35 mmHg, a mean gradient of 11 mmHg, and a valve area of 0.96 cm^2. Cardiac CT showed mitral annular calcification from one trigone to the other along the posterior annulus. Evaluation of the coronary arteries revealed no obstructive lesions and showed a right dominant system. You have recommended mitral valve replacement, Maze procedure, and left atrial appendage amputation.

You proceed with a trans-septal incision and place a purse string around the ostium of the coronary sinus, inserting just the tip of the retrograde cardioplegia cannula for better biventricular protection as you anticipate a longer case. Before proceeding with the mitral valve repair, you amputate the left atrial appendage and oversew the left atrial appendage stump with two layers of running 4–0 prolene suture. The mitral valve is heavily calcified with severe posterior mitral annular calcification. Considering your options either to simply drive needles around or through the calcium for the most radical approach you resign yourself to resecting the calcium with a plan to resurface the ventricle. Fortunately, the majority of the calcium is located in the posterior aspect of the annulus itself with limited extension

A. Kreso · S. I. Melnitchouk (✉)
Department of Surgery, Massachusetts General Hospital, Boston, MA, USA
e-mail: smelnitchouk@mgh.harvard.edu

A. Kreso
e-mail: akreso@mgh.harvard.edu

© The Author(s), under exclusive license to Springer Nature Switzerland AG 2022   143
T. M. Sundt et al. (eds.), *Near Misses in Cardiac Surgery*,
https://doi.org/10.1007/978-3-030-92750-9_36

into the ventricle. You reconstruct the posterior annulus with a pericardial patch, reinforced the medial annulus with Gore-Tex neocords from 3 stumps of the papillary muscles and secure a 27 mm bioprosthetic valve. The valve sits well, and you are satisfied with the patch repair. You close the left atriotomy and hold your breath as the patient weans off bypass [2].

Much to your relief, no blood emanates from the atrioventricular groove. You've seen that rush of red blood appear before between the heart and the diaphragm and hope never to see it again. There is, however, troublesome bleeding coming from behind and lateral to the pulmonary artery. As you examine the suture lines, you notice a large leak at the posterior aspect of the left atrial appendage closure line. You wonder why your cardiology colleagues seem to think fiddling with the appendage is a benign endeavor as you search to localize the bleeding to place a repair stitch. You gently lift and rotate the heart just enough to bring the suture line into view. Much to your delight you manage to place a pledgeted repair stitch in just the right spot, which controls the bleeding from the left atrial amputation site. Happy with the repair, you slowly return the heart down into the chest. Your sense of accomplishment is short-lived. Much to your chagrin, there is now bright red blood pooling from the back of the heart. It is clear that the atrial appendage is no longer the culprit.

Solution

You ask the perfusion team to go back on bypass, and once flow is established, you cross clamp the aorta and give antegrade and retrograde cardioplegia. You are now certain the culprit is AV groove disruption after the MAC debridement. Once you have re-arrested the heart, you re-open the atriotomy and examine the mitral valve. Unable to identify any problem, you confirm that the left atrial appendage amputation suture line is competent. After you remove the bioprosthesis and examine the patch repair area, you find the patch reconstruction has torn through the tissue causing a resultant defect in the left corner of the patch. You sew another patch to cover the defect and reinforce the entire new suture line to the left ventricle with a series of pledgeted sutures. You were careful at the initial repair to preserve segments of anterior leaflet with chordal attachments to reinforce your repair. This time you place them strategically to cover the area of tear. Once again you replace the valve. Although an intraaortic balloon pump is inserted to further unload the left ventricle, you are able to come off bypass on moderate inotropic support. You gently pack around the heart, leaving the chest open. After two days, the chest is closed, the IABP is removed, and you are relieved to have no further issues with bleeding. The patient is extubated on day 6 and leaves the hospital on postoperative day 14. You are relieved the patient has survived this devastating complication and have a new perspective on whether every left atrial appendage should be amputated, even if indicated.

Discussion

AV dissociation can be diagnosed after coming off cardiopulmonary bypass or soon after the procedure. The massive intrapericardial hemorrhage can be a lethal event. The repair for this defect is to secure a pericardial patch over the area of perforation using a running prolene suture, which may be subsequently reinforced with interrupted pledgeted sutures placed in a horizontal mattress fashion. The best approach is to avoid the problem altogether. For this reason, when extensive calcium is encountered, one may opt *not* to amputate the atrial appendage to avoid the potentially disastrous consequences associated with manipulating a heart that has extensive MAC. Alternatively, the appendage may be closed using a patch from within or by primary closure from within, using a purse string or in linear fashion, but this is notoriously unreliable and carries significant risk of re-canalization [3]. The appendage can be also excluded from the outside with several pledgeted stitches or a commercially available clip. Regardless, meticulous attention must be paid to avoid lifting the heart after any operation involving mitral valve replacement, such as revising a distal anastomosis on an obtuse marginal branch after removing the cross clamp.

When debriding calcium that is encountered in the sub-annular space, the principle is to resect only that amount necessary to place the valve and facilitate suture placement. This is especially important when there is extensive calcium that crosses onto the ventricular side as this increases the risk for AV groove disruption. When extensive calcium is resected, it is imperative that the pericardial patch straddles the annulus and covers the entire area of decalcification. The patch should be secured by placing the sutures into healthy myocardium for a tension-free repair with careful placement of sutures near the coronary vessels. One should also attempt to perform a chordal-sparing valve replacement for additional chordal support in the area of the left ventricular suture line. Even if the best technique is achieved, there is some residual risk of AV groove disruption particularly when the heart is manipulated after an annular patch repair. As this case illustrates, fixing a bleeding site on the posterior aspect of the heart can be challenging and result in AV groove disruption.

An alternate approach is to place a large teflon felt "gasket" between the sewing ring of the valve and the annulus. After seating the valve one then tacks the peripheral edge of the patch to the left atrial wall for added protection against paravalvular leaks. While some surgeons argue simply to drive the valve suture needles though the calcium, this can lead to late paravalvular leak.

Bibliography

1. Carpentier A, Adams D, Filsoufi F. Carpentier's reconstructive valve surgery. 1st ed. Maryland Heights, Mo; Saunders/Elsevier, copyright; 2010.
2. Feindel CM, Tufail Z, David TE, Ivanov J, Armstrong S. Mitral valve surgery in patients with extensive calcification of the mitral annulus. J Thorac Cardiovasc Surg. 2003;126:777–82.
3. Kanderian AS, Gillinov MV, Pettersson GB, Blackstone E, Klein AL. Success of surgical left atrial appendage closure: assessment by Transesophageal Echocardiography. JACC. 2008;52 (11):924–9.
4. Bedeir K, Kaneko T, Aranki S. Current and evolving strategies in the management of severe mitral annular calcification. J Thorac Cardiovasc Surg. 2019;157:555–66.
5. Hussain ST, Idrees J, Brozzi NA, Blackstone EH, Pettersson GB. Use of annulus washer after debridement: a new mitral valve replacement technique for patients with severe mitral annular calcification. J Thorac Cardiovasc Surg. 2013;145(6):1672–4. https://doi.org/10.1016/j.jtcvs. 2012.12.049 PMID: 23679966.

Chapter 37
Options for a Patient with History of HITT

Jenna Cottral and Kenneth T. Shelton

Problem

The ventricular assist device practice at your institution has grown dramatically since the recent recruitment of an enthusiastic medical director with connections to the community to attract patients with heart failure. You have learned that while the results can be dramatic, so are the complications. You are beginning to see things you might never have imagined possible. Today a patient for whom you inserted a left ventricular assist device (LVAD) 6 months ago is now in the emergency room. She is 51 years old with a terrible family history of premature coronary artery disease. About 6 months ago she underwent coronary artery bypass but was unable to wean from bypass. She suffered a prolonged course including ECMO support before HeartMate III (LVAD) insertion, as well as antibody-confirmed heparin-induced thrombocytopenia (HIT) and thrombosis (HITT) with an optical density (OD) of 3.1, which was diagnosed after thrombosis of her left common femoral artery and right internal jugular vein. She was eventually discharged on warfarin and has done remarkably well until today, when multiple low-flow alarms sounded at home.

In the ED, a CT scan demonstrates a large anterior mediastinal hematoma with mass effect on the right ventricle concerning for tamponade physiology, as well as apparent separation of the outflow cannula from the body of the LVAD! She has become progressively hemodynamically unstable in the emergency room and your resident asks if he should book an emergent chest exploration with possible LVAD revision. You agree and turn to your anesthesia colleagues to discuss options for systemic anticoagulation on cardiopulmonary bypass given her history of HITT and no recent antibody serology.

J. Cottral · K. T. Shelton (✉)
Department of Anesthesia, Massachusetts General Hospital, Boston, MA, USA
e-mail: kshelton@mgh.harvard.edu

J. Cottral
e-mail: Jennifer.cottral@mgh.harvard.edu

© The Author(s), under exclusive license to Springer Nature Switzerland AG 2022   147
T. M. Sundt et al. (eds.), *Near Misses in Cardiac Surgery*,
https://doi.org/10.1007/978-3-030-92750-9_37

Solution

Your anesthesia colleagues reassure you that heparin will be safe during bypass despite the patient's history of HITT. First, they argue, HITT is a stoichiometric-dependent phenomenon and the large doses of heparin used in bypass will overwhelm the present antibody's formation of heparin-PF4 complexes. Second, the median time to antibody clearance is 50 days for platelet activation assays and 85 to 90 days for immunoassays and thus, at 6 months since HITT diagnosis, it is unlikely that the patient currently has circulating anti-PF4/heparin antibodies. Third, complete heparin reversal with protamine is possible after weaning off bypass which will decrease the likelihood of seroconversion from heparin re-exposure. You and your anesthesia colleagues agree to use heparin for the case. While you have confidence in the logic of your course, you are no less grateful when the patient does well perioperatively.

Discussion

Heparin-induced thrombocytopenia (HIT) and thrombosis (HITT) is an immune phenomenon provoked by inflammation or infection leading to the formation of antibodies against the heparin–platelet factor 4 (PF4) complex, which in turn activates platelets leading to thrombocytopenia and thrombosis. HIT/HITT is a clinical diagnosis often made by a high pre-test probability of HIT/HITT by the 4-T score, a positive antibody test by enzyme-linked immunoassay with a high optical density (OD) and a positive functional assay. Non-operating room management of HIT/HITT includes discontinuation of heparin and initiation of a non-heparin anticoagulant at therapeutic-intensity dosing, with guidelines recommending either argatroban, bivalirudin, danaparoid, fondaparinux, or a direct oral anticoagulant. Screening for asymptomatic deep vein thrombosis (DVT) by compression ultra-sonography is recommended in the bilateral lower extremities, as well as any upper extremity with an indwelling central venous catheter. However, anticoagulation at therapeutic-intensity dosing should continue until platelet recovery even in the absence of DVT. In patients who require cardiovascular surgery with acute HIT or subacute HIT with normal platelet count but positive immune and functional assays (subacute HIT A), current guidelines recommend that surgery be delayed if possible until the functional assay is negative (subacute HIT B) and/or if both the functional and immune assays are negative (remote HIT). If surgical delay is not possible, the guidelines suggest intraoperative anticoagulation should be achieved either with a direct thrombin inhibitor (bivalirudin/argatroban) or heparin. If the decision is made to use heparin, the team should also consider treatment with plasma exchange or heparin in combination with a potent antiplatelet agent. Argatroban may also be used instead of bivalirudin in patients with renal failure requiring renal replacement therapy. Heparin can be used for patients with subacute HIT B or remote HIT, but only in the intraoperative period, and heparin should be avoided both pre- and postoperatively. Postoperative platelet count should be closely monitored for any patient with a history of HIT who received intraoperative heparin because delayed-onset (autoimmune) HIT has been described, usually occurring 5 to 10 days after the intraoperative heparin exposure.

Bibliography

1. Arepally G. Heparin-induced thrombocytopenia. Blood. 2017;129(21):2864–72.
2. Cuker A, Arepally GM, Chong BH, Cines DB, Greunacher A, Gruel Y, Linkins LA, Rodner SB, Selleng S, Warkentin TE, Wex A, Mustafa RA, Morgan RL, Santesso N. American Society of Hematology 2018 guidelines for management of venous thromboembolism: heparin-induced thrombocytopenia. Blood Adv. 2018;2(22):3360–92.
3. Shore-Lesserson L, Baker RA, Ferraris VA, Greilich PE, Fitzgerald D, Roman P, Hammon JW. The society of thoracic surgeons, The society of cardiovascular anesthesiologists, and The American society of extracorporeal technology: clinical practice guidelines anticoagulation during cardiopulmonary bypass. Anesth Analg. 2018;126(2):413–24.

Chapter 38
Ventricular Dysrhythmia after AVR

Andrew C. W. Baldwin and Thoralf Sundt

Problem

As you enter the callback number into your phone, you are curious yet apprehensive. You have a message that reads *"give me a call, I'd like to chat"* sent by the newly appointed director of the cardiac catheterization lab—a prominent cardiologist with a national reputation with whom you have only spoken in passing. After some initial pleasantries, he reveals that his mother has severe aortic stenosis. Of course, he initially pushed for her to have a transcatheter valve replacement, but despite his forceful influence she was nervously declined by a multidisciplinary committee reluctant to overlook not only her diminutive and tortuous femoral vessels, but also her bicuspid disease and low-riding coronary ostia. You are humbled to hear that your reputation has grown such that you were the surgeon recommended for surgical valve replacement.

You review her imaging and confirm her stenotic bicuspid valve with mild associated aortic insufficiency. She is 78 years old with no other comorbidities. Her coronaries are free of significant disease, her ventricular function is normal, and her BSA of 1.7 m^2 is a far outlier amongst your referrals. A chance to impress an important audience with a routine AVR? You consider buying a lottery ticket on your way home.

After an uneventful sternotomy and initiation of cardiopulmonary bypass, you cross clamp, administer antegrade cardioplegia down the root, and open the aorta to find a heavily calcified bicuspid valve. At first you think her small aorta is limiting your view, but you debride the annulus to confirm that a #21 valve sizer will just

A. C. W. Baldwin
Division of Cardiac Surgery, Straub Medical Center, Honolulu, HI, USA
e-mail: Andrew.Baldwin@hphmg.org

T. Sundt (✉)
Division of Cardiac Surgery, Massachusetts General Hospital, Boston, MA, USA
e-mail: tsundt@mgh.harvard.edu

© The Author(s), under exclusive license to Springer Nature Switzerland AG 2022   151
T. M. Sundt et al. (eds.), *Near Misses in Cardiac Surgery*,
https://doi.org/10.1007/978-3-030-92750-9_38

barely squeeze in. Having already cross-checked her BSA with the manufacturer guidelines before scrubbing in, you quietly exhale and call for a 21 mm bioprosthetic valve knowing it will be of sufficient size (just). You carefully maneuver the prosthesis through a tight sinotubular junction and take your time seating each knot given the difficulty of reaching the sewing ring within the small root. Despite these challenges, the valve goes in quickly, and you close the aortotomy and release the cross-clamp.

Transesophageal echo shows a well-seated well-functioning valve without paravalvular leak. Several minutes later, the anesthesiologist points out some ST changes in leads II, III, and aVF, and you shake your head as you admit you could have done a better job de-airing the root had you not been distracted by trying to avoid a second dose of cardioplegia. After a few minutes with higher perfusion pressures, the EKG normalizes and feeling reassured, you proceed with decannulation. You call for the wires, reminding yourself to make them look stylish for when her son inevitably checks the post-op films. Just then, her pressures drop precipitously, and she goes into a ventricular tachycardia. Reality hits, and you call for the wire cutters.

Solution

You immediately suspect a problem with the right coronary artery. The anesthesiologists had not yet pulled the echo probe, and now report new inferior wall hypokinesis and right ventricular dysfunction. Concerned about potential ischemia, you quickly re-open, heparinize, and re-cannulate for bypass. Upon direct inspection, the RV appears dilated and hypokinetic. Immediately following institution of bypass, the inferior-lead ST elevations begin to resolve. Concerned that the ostium of the right coronary is being obstructed by the bioprosthetic valve strut, you proceed with construction of a bypass graft to the RCA. You explore the right thigh and find a reasonable-appearing segment of saphenous vein that you excise, de-branch, and reverse. Seeking to avoid arresting the heart again, you identify the proximal RCA and place silastic tapes proximally and distally to the area most suitable for bypass. You open the vessel longitudinally to find marginal antegrade flow as you perform your distal anastomosis. Calling for perfusion to reduce their bypass flow, you then apply a partial occluding clamp to the ascending aorta and perform your proximal anastomosis. After ample reperfusion time, you wean from bypass and confirm a return to normal biventricular function. You again decannulate and call for the wires, a bit less giddy than the first time around.

Discussion

Coronary obstruction from a prosthetic valve strut is a rare but well-documented phenomenon capable of causing acute decompensation from myocardial ischemia. The valve posts of a stented bioprosthesis can be challenging to properly position within a narrow aortic root, and bicuspid valves (as was the case with this patient) are more commonly associated with anomalous coronary ostia. In addition, the engineering employed to optimize orifice area of the current prostheses has required displacement of the actual valve leaflet attachments a bit above the sewing ring, creating a "rail" even at the nadirs of the prostheses which can be obstructive to low lying coronaries. With the preoperative discovery of a small root, bicuspid valve, and low-riding coronary arteries during TAVR evaluation, your patient was clearly at higher risk for this complication.

The initial discovery of inferior lead ST changes (though transient) was the harbinger of a larger surgical complication. Several scenarios can present in a similar fashion. Air traveling down the RCA (your initial assumption) is common due to the anterior takeoff of the right ostium and typically results in transient ST changes. Embolic debris, coronary dissection from instrumentation including osteal cardioplegia cannulae, suture ligation (particularly of an aberrant circumflex originating in the right coronary sinus), and obstruction of the coronary ostium should also be considered. The presence of a small aortic root should lead to a higher index of suspicion for any coronary pathology.

Aortic root enlargement may have prevented this complication. Extension of the aortotomy toward the midpoint of the non-coronary cusp allows for better visualization of the root during implantation and reduces the potential for patient-prosthesis mismatch. A tongue of bovine pericardium allows for enlargement of the root during closure of the aortotomy and can prevent drawing the RCA ostium up against the rail or commissural post that can be difficult to appreciate with the root open.

Quick recognition of this complication and accepting its reality is essential to avoid prolonged ischemia. Re-establishment of cardiopulmonary bypass reduces myocardial demand and will help stabilize the patient. Open saphenous vein harvesting is the fastest conduit choice and will immediately provide high flow. The distal anastomosis should be to the proximal or mid RCA, not distally to the PDA as one needs to provide adequate perfusion of the acute marginal branches. Given the ischemic hit to the right ventricle, the bypass should be performed without re-arresting the heart if possible. Replacing the valve or performing a root enlargement at this time would dramatically increase the complexity of the surgery while prolonging ischemic time and would likely result in postoperative right heart failure.

Bibliography

1. Salerno TA, Bergsland J, Calafiore AM, Cordell AR, Kon ND, Bhayana JN. Acute right ventricular failure during aortic valvular operation due to mechanical problem in the right coronary artery. Ann Thorac Surg. 1996;61:706–7.
2. Grubb KJ. Aortic root enlargement during aortic valve replacement: Nicks and Manouguian Techniques. Op Tech Thorac Cardiovasc Surg. 2016;20:206–18.
3. Nicks R, Cartmill T, Bernstein L. Hypoplasia of the aortic root: the problem of aortic valve replacement. Thorax. 1970;25(3):339–46.
4. Manouguian S, Seybold-Epting W. Patch enlargement of the aortic valve ring by extending the aortic incision into the anterior mitral leaflet: new operative technique. J Thorac Cardiovasc Surg. 1979;78(3):402–12.
5. Dhareshwar J, Sundt TM, et al. Aortic root enlargement: what are the operative risks? J Thorac Cardiovasc Surg. 2007;134(4):916–24.

Chapter 39
Postoperative Hypoxemia

Rachel Steinhorn and Michael G. Fitzsimons

Problem

It's another glorious night in the operating room, and you have just finished an emergent valve sparing root and proximal aortic arch replacement under deep hypothermic circulatory arrest for a type A aortic dissection in a 42-year-old man with Marfan's disease. Time under circulatory arrest was 19 min, with an even 180 min spent on cardiopulmonary bypass. The patient flew off bypass after his initial hypovolemia was repleted with a liter of salvaged autologous blood and two units of packed red blood cells. The last of the protamine went in five minutes ago and an activated coagulation time is within normal limits with zero heparin remaining, but the patient continues to ooze diffusely from tissue beds. After discussion with the anesthesia team, two units of fresh frozen plasma and a unit of platelets are transfused empirically while awaiting the results of coagulation labs. You begin to achieve better hemostasis and proceed to close.

After sternal closure, you scrub out to let your fellow finish the educational job of skin suturing and dressing. It's at this point that the attending anesthesiologist informs you they're having difficulty with oxygenation. The pervasive beeping from the anesthesia side of the drapes suddenly strikes you as more cacophonous than usual. A glance at the monitors shows that SpO_2 is 89%, central venous pressure is 8 mmHg, pulmonary artery pressure 32/14 mmHg, and blood pressure 102/55 mmHg. Cardiac output by thermodilution is 5.5 L/min with an index of 3.3 $L/min/m^2$. As you consider your options, the pulse oximeter continues its mournful downward trend in a discordant duel with the ventilator alarming high plateau

R. Steinhorn · M. G. Fitzsimons (✉)
Division of Cardiac Anesthesia, Department of Anesthesia, Critical Care, and Pain Medicine, Massachusetts General Hospital, Boston, MA, USA
e-mail: mfitzsimons@mgh.harvard.edu

R. Steinhorn
e-mail: rsteinhorn@mgh.harvard.edu

© The Author(s), under exclusive license to Springer Nature Switzerland AG 2022
T. M. Sundt et al. (eds.), *Near Misses in Cardiac Surgery*,
https://doi.org/10.1007/978-3-030-92750-9_39

pressures of 38 cm H_2O. An arterial blood gas returns with pH 7.36, $PaCO_2$ 43, PaO_2 87 on FiO_2 100%. You didn't expect your cardiac surgery to be derailed by a pulmonary problem, but nevertheless, it looks like your night isn't done yet. Frustrated you mumble "in with the good air and out with the bad." How hard can it be?

Solution

Many roads lead to hypoxemia, and you set to work with the anesthesia team to narrow your differential diagnosis as you treat. You return to the fundamental ABC's: Is this a problem with the airway, or with effective ventilation and oxygenation? Delivery of oxygen from a wall source is confirmed on the ventilator screen. The mechanical ventilator circuit has no obstructed tubing, ruling that out as the cause of high airway pressures. A quick fiberoptic bronchoscopy confirms that the endotracheal tube is 3 cm above the carina with no kinking or blockage by a mucus plug to increase airway resistance. Frothy secretions are suctioned from otherwise clear segmental bronchi with no evidence of sanguineous fluid concerning for diffuse alveolar hemorrhage in the setting of coagulopathy.

With an airway obstruction swiftly ruled out, you focus on problems of ventilation and gas exchange. Bronchodilators are administered with no improvement. The expiratory CO_2 waveform is not the ominous shark fin of an obstructed exhalation, and the anesthesiologist reports that the increase in both peak and plateau pressures is more consistent with a change in parenchymal compliance rather than bronchospasm. Transesophageal echocardiography (TEE) confirms that biventricular function is normal with no aortic or mitral regurgitation and there is no pleural effusion, though the lungs appear so consolidated bilaterally they resemble the liver. No new atrial or ventricular septal defect is visualized, and concern for shunt is low. The patient remains hemodynamically stable on norepinephrine 4 mcg/min (0.05mcg/kg/min) throughout.

You strongly suspect a noncardiogenic source of acute pulmonary edema. Whether it is transfusion associated lung injury (TRALI), which is a reasonable suspicion given the timing, or acute respiratory distress syndrome (ARDS) secondary to cardiopulmonary bypass, or a combination of both makes little difference. The treatment remains the same. You discuss optimizing mechanical ventilation for lung protection with the anesthesia team, which reduces tidal volumes from 8 cc/kg to 6 cc/kg predicted body weight and increases the respiratory rate to 28 breaths/min to maintain minute ventilation. A recruitment maneuver and decremental PEEP trial is performed to reduce atelectasis following bypass and to maximize alveoli available for gas exchange. Although you know it may not improve mortality or morbidity, the patient's persistent hypoxemia prompts you to initiate inhaled nitric oxide. You notify the hospital blood bank and set aside the products transfused for later anti-HLA antibody testing to further work up TRALI. After pulmonary vasodilator initiation, the subsequent ABG improves to pH 7.35, $PaCO_2$ 48, PaO_2 107 on FiO_2 100%, and you transfer the patient to the intensive care unit in stable condition.

Discussion

In this case, the broad differential diagnosis of hypoxemia is rapidly narrowed to a problem of oxygen diffusion, likely ARDS secondary to cardiopulmonary bypass and/or TRALI. Airway obstruction, hypoventilation, and inadequate oxygen delivery are effectively ruled out through assessment of the mechanical ventilator and bronchoscopy. Other potential etiologies of ventilation/perfusion mismatch after cardiac surgery, such as new intracardiac shunt, are less likely given the absence of findings on TEE. Similarly, cardiogenic pulmonary edema or transfusion-associated circulatory overload is less concerning with normal biventricular function by TEE and a normal cardiac output calculated by the PA line.

ARDS is a frequent cause of hypoxemic respiratory failure characterized by poor lung compliance in the setting of noncardiogenic pulmonary and inflammatory alveolar damage. Cardiopulmonary bypass increases the risk of ARDS both by activation of the systemic inflammatory cascade and by increasing intrapulmonary shunt secondary to atelectasis. Observational studies find that 67–87% of patients develop mild ARDS by clinical criteria (PaO_2:FiO_2 < 300) after cardiopulmonary bypass, and 20–30% of patients have moderate ARDS (PaO_2:FiO_2 < 200).

Likewise, TRALI is a pulmonary transfusion reaction diagnosed by the development of acute, noncardiogenic pulmonary edema within six hours of receiving a transfusion. Donor leukocyte antibodies bind to recipient antigens, precipitating neutrophil activation and pulmonary sequestration that triggers the inflammatory cascade, disrupts the alveolar-capillary barrier, and causes inflammatory pulmonary edema. Recipient risk factors for TRALI include emergency cardiac surgery, hematologic malignancy, massive transfusion, sepsis, mechanical ventilation, longer cardiopulmonary bypass times, and a high APACHE II score. TRALI has been reported with all blood products, but components with a higher plasma volume (fresh frozen plasma, whole blood, apheresis platelet concentrates) represent the highest risk. Multiparous female donors have a higher risk of developing HLA or HNA antibodies and are associated with a higher likelihood of recipient TRALI. In this respect, the histopathological manifestation of TRALI is similar to ARDS, which makes differentiating between the two difficult when patients have risk factors for both.

Fortunately, the treatment is identical: Supportive care to maintain oxygenation while reducing the risk of further ventilator-induced lung injury. Lung protective mechanical ventilation should be maintained with tidal volumes 6–8 cm^3/kg predicted body weight, plateau pressures < 35 mmHg, and positive end expiratory pressure > 5 mmHg to prevent atelectasis. The mortality benefit of neuromuscular blockade has been called into question by negative results from recent randomized controlled trials, but still recommended to maintain patient-ventilator synchrony in moderate-to-severe ARDS. Prone positioning improves mortality in moderate-to-severe ARDS but is relatively contraindicated in the setting of cardiac surgery via sternotomy. In severe hypoxemia refractory to ventilator optimization and supplemental treatments, the use of venovenous extracorporeal membrane oxygenation is supported as a rescue therapy.

Bibliography

1. Voelker MT, Spieth P. Blood transfusion associated lung injury. J Thorac Dis. 2019;11 (8):3609–15.
2. McVey MJ, Kapur R, Cserti-Gazdewich C, Semple JW, Karkouti K, Kuebler WM. Transfusion-related acute lung injury in the perioperative patient. Anesthesiology. 2019;131 (3):693–715.
3. Rong LQ, Di Franco A, Gaudino M. Acute respiratory distress syndrome after cardiac surgery. J Thorac Dis. 2016;8(10):E1177–86.
4. Papazian L, Aubron C, Brochard L, et al. Formal guidelines: management of acute respiratory distress syndrome. Ann Intensive Care. 2019;9:69.
5. Munshi L, Walkey A, Goligher E, Pham T, Uleryk EM, Fan E. Venovenous extracorporeal membrane oxygenation for acute respiratory distress syndrome: a systematic review and meta-analysis. Lancet Respir Med. 2019;7(2):163–72.
6. Dijkhuizen A, De Bruin R, Arbous S. Incidence, risk factors and outcome of TRALI after cardiac surgery. Crit Care. 2013;17(Suppl 2):P373. https://doi.org/10.1186/cc12311.

Chapter 40
Orthotopic Heart Transplant (OHT) after LVAD

S. Alireza Rabi and David A. D'Alessandro

Problem

You are about to head home after a long day in the operating room, when the transplant coordinator at your center calls to inform you of an offer for a heart for one of your long-term heart failure patients. Mr. S has had a left ventricular assist (LVAD) device as a bridge-to-transplant for 18 months. His pulmonary artery pressures, which were concerningly high at the time of LAVD insertion, have come down to a tolerable range and are not likely to fall further. During the last few months, he has had multiple admissions to the hospital for GI bleeds, and during his last office visit with you, he confides that, demoralized by the frequent admissions, he is really looking forward to a more permanent solution. After determining the heart would be a good match for Mr. S, you inform him of the offer and he gladly accepts! That night he is taken to the OR for an orthotropic heart transplant.

As the result of significant adhesions from his previous cardiac surgeries (mitral valve repair, coronary bypass surgery, and most recently, the LVAD placement), the explant is challenging, but by the time the donor's heart is in the room, you are ready to perform the anastomosis. You perform a bicaval anastomosis as usual. The implant is notable for a size mismatch between the donor and the SVC diameter, but you are not overly concerned as it is common for the native SVC to have a significantly larger diameter. The donor was a healthy 28-year-old, almost half Mr. S's age. After completing the anastomosis and removing the cross-clamp, you are gratified when the heart begins to beat immediately and vigorously. Next, you divert your attention to hemostasis, and after a few repair sutures, you are satisfied. You are able wean Mr. S from cardiopulmonary bypass initially, but the hemo-

S. A. Rabi · D. A. D'Alessandro (✉)
Department of Surgery, Massachusetts General Hospital, Boston, MA, USA
e-mail: dadalessandro@mgh.harvard.edu

S. A. Rabi
e-mail: srabi@mgh.harvard.edu

© The Author(s), under exclusive license to Springer Nature Switzerland AG 2022   159
T. M. Sundt et al. (eds.), *Near Misses in Cardiac Surgery*,
https://doi.org/10.1007/978-3-030-92750-9_40

dynamic parameters deteriorate within a few minutes. The mean arterial pressure (MAP) is low and by TEE the left ventricle is underfilled. Right ventricular failure seems the most likely explanation, not an uncommon complication in transplantation, particularly when there are concerns about pulmonary hypertension. But the pulmonary artery pressures are also down as is the CVP, and by ECHO as well as visual inspection of the heart, the RV is hyperdynamic. Systemic vasodilatation is a possibility as well, but the cardiac index is also low. If you were not already gowned and gloved, you would scratch your head as you ponder the possibilities. What is going on?

Just then the anesthesiologist asks you if they can put the patient in a reverse Trendelenburg position because the head looks swollen. The penny drops: you know immediately there is a technical problem and inform the room that you will need to re-initiate full CPB support.

Solution

You re-establish CPB, snare the cavae, and take down the SVC anastomosis. No need to cross clamp the aorta and re-arrest the heart since it is the right side you are addressing. You revise the anastomosis, this time trimming the donor SVC lower down closer to the SVC-RA junction, spatulating it posteriorly away from the SA node. Using triangulation technique and smaller bites, you perform an anastomosis that would make Alexis Carrel proud! You consider performing a "locking suture" to prevent purse stringing the anastomosis when tying but decide to perform your usual technique instead. This time you wean the patient from bypass without any difficulty. The RV pressures are within the normal range, and the upper extremity swelling has improved. You are happy to observe that the patient has normal sinus rhythm, since one consequence of excessive manipulation of the SVC-RA junction is damage to the SA node or the supplying artery.

Discussion

Low cardiac output state with low RV pressures, a hyperdynamic heart, and swollen head indicate SVC narrowing leading to low preload. Stricture of the SVC anastomosis is a rare complication of the bicaval technique. The most common risk factor is donor-recipient mismatch. Many heart transplant recipients have elevated central venous pressures that can manifest in vena cava enlargement. Significant mismatch between the donor and recipient and large bites taken at the SVC anastomosis site can lead to stricture.

If suspicion is high, this is much better addressed immediately. Late postoperative treatment of SVC syndrome is possible percutaneously with stenting but is far from trivial given the frequent need to access the transplanted heart for endocardial biopsies. A wise surgeon is remembered to have said "if you leave the operating room unhappy, you will be back unhappy." Best to fix the problem now.

Bibliography

1. Sze DY, Robbins RC, Semba CP, Razavi MK, Dake MD. Superior vena cava syndrome after heart transplantation: percutaneous treatment of a complication of bicaval anastomoses. J Thorac Cardiovasc Surg. 1998;116(2):253–61. https://doi.org/10.1016/S0022-5223(98)70124-2.
2. Sachdeva R, Seib PM, Burns SA, Fontenot EE, Frazier EA. Stenting for superior vena cava obstruction in pediatric heart transplant recipients. Catheter Cardiovasc Interv. 2007;70(6):888–92. https://doi.org/10.1002/ccd.21296.

Chapter 41
Postoperative Infection

Myles E. Lee and Thoralf M. Sundt

Problem

A 73-year-old diabetic patient with a strong family history of coronary artery disease presents with a 1-year history of exertional angina. Cardiac catheterization reveals inferobasal akinesis, an 80% left main lesion, a 95% diagonal lesion, and total obstruction of the right coronary artery.

At surgery, you find a surprisingly large transmural infarction involving most of the posterior and inferior walls of the right and left ventricles. You graft the left internal thoracic artery to the left anterior descending and construct vein grafts to the diagonal, circumflex, and posterior descending coronary arteries. You separate the patient from cardiopulmonary bypass on moderate inotropic support and transfer him to the cardiac surgical intensive care unit in satisfactory condition. The patient is extubated on postoperative day 1 and weaned from inotropes on day 2. Later that evening, the patient spikes to 101.6 °F. You obtain blood, sputum, and urine cultures. During this time, you notice a low systemic vascular resistance with labile blood pressure as well as oliguria and rising serum creatinine, for which you start a dopamine drip. By the morning of the third postoperative day the patient requires reintubation for acute respiratory failure. Because of left lower lobe atelectasis, you perform a bronchoscopy to rule out a mucus plug. During the bronchoscopy, after a cough, you notice a small amount of serosanguineous drainage in the lower third of a totally benign-appearing sternotomy incision. It is less

M. E. Lee
Department of Cardiothoracic Surgery, Centinela Hospital Medical Center, Inglewood, CA, USA

T. M. Sundt (✉)
Division of Cardiac Surgery, Massachusetts General Hospital, Boston, MA, USA
e-mail: tsundt@mgh.harvard.edu

© The Author(s), under exclusive license to Springer Nature Switzerland AG 2022
T. M. Sundt et al. (eds.), *Near Misses in Cardiac Surgery*,
https://doi.org/10.1007/978-3-030-92750-9_41

than 72 h after a completely uneventful operation and this patient now challenges you with his imminent self-destruction, making a cruel mockery of your best efforts. What should you do now?

Solution

You obtain a Gram stain of the sternal drainage and are shocked to find it reveals numerous gram-negative bacteria. Simultaneously, you learn that the blood cultures from the previous evening have grown out a gram-negative rod as well. The patient's white blood cell count has risen from 8,900 on the first postoperative evening to over 14,000. You start antibiotics and return the patient to the operating room without delay.

At surgery, you identify purulent material in the mediastinum and an acute fibrinous peel over the heart, as well as a 500 cm^3 purulent effusion in the left pleural space. You irrigate the mediastinum, pericardium, and pleural space with 6 L of saline and place a new pleural tube. The bone appears intact; however, given evidence of deep infection you elect to place a negative pressure wound treatment (NPWT) device and return to the OR in 48 h to reassess. The patient defervesces and at re-exploration you elect to reclose the sternum with wires, reapproximate the fascia, and close the skin with interrupted vertical mattress sutures.

Discussion

The incidence of postoperative mediastinitis in the current era has fallen to less than 1%, which is remarkable given the increasing number of co-morbidities in our patients. When it occurs, however, it is associated with significant morbidity and diminished long-term survival. Although the etiology in this case was never identified, the rapid, almost ferocious, onset in this relatively healthy patient was consistent with a significant bacterial inoculation at the time of surgery or in the intensive care unit. Possible sources include contamination of the monitoring lines and injection ports, the injectate used to measure thermal dilution cardiac outputs, the anesthesia circuit, the perfusion lines, or the surgical instruments.

Other causes may predispose to this complication, including advanced age, poor nutritional status, diabetes mellitus, pre-existing but subclinical infection, impaired immunocompetence, prolonged duration of surgery, low cardiac output, emergency reoperation for bleeding, use of both internal thoracic arteries for bypass conduits, and break in surgical technique. This patient's survival was a direct function of his otherwise excellent condition, the rapidity of the diagnosis, and the aggressive treatment from the beginning of his illness.

In the early days of cardiac surgery, the treatment of mediastinitis consisted of debridement, open drainage, and packing with slow granulation of the open wound over a period of weeks to months. Subsequently, a practice of sternal rewiring and mediastinal irrigation with dilute povidone iodine solution was adopted; however, exceedingly high systemic iodine levels have been demonstrated, risking renal dysfunction, thyroid dysfunction, and electrolyte abnormalities. Irrigation with dilute antibiotic solution is an alternative although data to support this practice are lacking. More popular today are negative pressure wound treatment (NPWT) devices. If the infection appears superficial without evidence of bony destruction, opening the skin and applying such a device may be helpful. If the infection is deep, it is critical to debride any necrotic tissue and "clean up" the wound before progressing to definitive closure. In this case, the bone appeared viable and was closed primarily; however, if there is bony destruction, aggressive debridement including removal of costal cartilage is essential before flap closure.

The best treatment of mediastinal infection, of course, is prevention. The most common cause of mediastinitis is *Staphylococcus aureus*. Accordingly, efforts specifically aimed at this organism have been shown to be effective, including both nasal disinfection with mupirocin and topical showering with chlorhexidine gluconate soap. Apart from these chemical interventions, the importance of sound surgical technique, including minimizing necrotic tissue necrosis due to overexuberant electrocautery and adequate mechanical closure of the sternum to eliminate motion, cannot be overemphasized. The patient's own status should be optimized preoperatively, including nutritional status, glycemic control and, if at all possible, smoking cessation. Current guidelines recommend perioperative antibiotics for 48 h.

Bibliography

1. Kaspersen AE, Nielsen SJ, Orrason AW, Petursdottir A, Sigurdsson MI, Jeppsson A, Gudbjartsson T. Short- and long-term mortality after deep sternal wound infection following cardiac surgery: experiences from SWEDEHEART. Eur J Cardiothorac Surg. 2021;60(2):233–41. https://doi.org/10.1093/ejcts/ezab080 PMID: 33623983.
2. Lazar HL, Vander Salm T, Engelman R, Orgill D, Gordon S. Prevention and management of sternal wound infections. J Thorac Cardiovasc Surg. 2016;152:962–72.
3. Mills C, Bryson P. The role of hyperbaric oxygen therapy in the treatment of sternal wound infection. Eur J Cardiothorac Surg. 2006;30(1):153–9. https://doi.org/10.1016/j.ejcts.2006.03.059 PMID: 16769519.
4. Gustafsson RI, Sjögren J, Ingemansson R. Deep sternal wound infection: a sternal-sparing technique with vacuum-assisted closure therapy. Ann Thorac Surg. 2003; 76(6):2048–53; discussion 2053. doi: https://doi.org/10.1016/s0003-4975(03)01337 PMID: 14667639

Chapter 42
Veno-venous ECMO

Travis Hull and Masaki Funamoto

Problem

An obese (BMI 44) 36-year-old man was admitted via the ED last evening with acute respiratory distress syndrome (ARDS) of uncertain etiology. His COVID-19 test is pending, but everyone is suspicious this is the cause. Three days ago he began having dyspnea. His respiratory status declined acutely before he could be admitted to the ICU requiring intubation and mechanical ventilation. Today, he began spiking fevers to as high as 102.5 F. Chest x-ray shows left lower lobe consolidation, and you suspect he has developed pneumonia. Broad spectrum antibiotics were initiated on admission, but it is already clear he will not tolerate pneumonia on top of his ARDS as his most recent blood gas demonstrates significant respiratory acidosis and worsening hypoxia despite optimal ventilator settings with high positive end expiratory pressure (PEEP). You book the OR to cannulate for veno-venous extracorporeal membrane oxygenation (VV-ECMO) as a bridge to recovery. The hybrid cardiac operating room facilitates transesophageal echocardiography (TEE) and fluoroscopy to monitor cannula insertion and confirm satisfactory cannula position. The patient is transported to the operating room as you turn to finish ICU rounds. Only minutes after he leaves the ICU on his way to the OR your pager goes off STAT: the patient has acutely decompensated while being bag masked during transport. Now you wish you had cannulated at the bedside! As you dash down the stairs you run through your options for emergent cannulation.

T. Hull · M. Funamoto (✉)
Department of Surgery, Massachusetts General Hospital, Boston, MA, USA
e-mail: Thull1@partners.org

M. Funamoto
Department of Cardiothoracic Surgery, Methodist Hospital, San Antonio, TX, USA

© The Author(s), under exclusive license to Springer Nature Switzerland AG 2022
T. M. Sundt et al. (eds.), *Near Misses in Cardiac Surgery*,
https://doi.org/10.1007/978-3-030-92750-9_42

The patient has likely decompensated from collapse of his non-complaint lungs in the setting of ARDS and obesity due to lack of PEEP during bag masking. The patient has an oxygen saturation in the 60 s and appears cyanotic. You prep and drape the patient from chin to knee and place a 4 Fr sheath in the right internal jugular vein (RIJ) under ultrasound guidance, as you plan to cannulate the patient using a dual lumen cannula reasoning that you will limit his duration of hypoxia by limiting procedure time and commencing VV-ECMO as quickly as possible. In the haste to arrive in the OR quickly, cardiac anesthesia has not had time to set up for TEE and the radiology technician has yet to prepare the equipment for fluoroscopy. Given the patient's critical status, you elect not to wait any longer. You call for a C-arm and begin advancing the wire via your 4 Fr sheath. The anesthesiologist places TEE probe in and you confirm that your wire advances across the RA and into the IVC. You sequentially dilate the tract to accommodate a dual lumen cannula for VV-ECMO but are informed by your colleagues in anesthesia that the patient is having runs of ventricular tachycardia. He is not going to tolerate this on top of profound hypoxia!

Solution

You suspect the wire has migrated from the IVC and is looping in the RV, which you confirm with fluoroscopy. Recognizing the significant risk of RV perforation when placing a dual lumen catheter in the emergent setting with limited image guidance, you elect to modify your approach. You retract your wire in the RIJ to the RA and instruct your senior fellow to place a 4 Fr sheath in the right femoral vein (RFV), as you will utilize bicaval cannulation via the RIJ and RFV. Single lumen VV-ECMO cannulas are uneventfully placed via the RIJ and RFV and their locations in the RA and IVC, respectively, are confirmed with TEE and fluoroscopy. The cannulas are connected to the ECMO circuit and VV-ECMO is commenced. You quickly achieve full flow and correct the patient's hypoxia and acidosis. The patient is returned to the cardiac surgery ICU where his COVID test has just returned negative. Managed on lung protective ventilator settings, he is decannulated from ECMO 5 days later and discharged from the hospital to rehab 2 weeks later after recovering from his ARDS.

Discussion

In this patient with non-compliant lungs from ARDS and morbid obesity who has a deteriorating respiratory status despite maximal vent settings and high PEEP, detachment from the mechanical ventilator for bag masking during transport is contra-indicated. His lungs, which are dependent on high end expiratory pressure, collapse once PEEP is removed and are unable to be recruited during emergent transfer to the OR [1]. Patients who are actively decompensating and will not tolerate transportation to the OR should be cannulated for VV-ECMO at the bedside so the patient can be provided with continuous PEEP while the cannulation procedure is carried out.

While a dual lumen cannula for VV-ECMO cannulation simplifies bedside care and permits ambulation, it should be avoided in the emergency setting. Placement of a dual lumen cannula is not trivial, and requires a controlled setting with optimal image guidance [2]. Imaging studies, such as TEE or/and fluoroscopy are required for real time visualization as a guide wire is placed and a cannula is advanced, even over a Super Stiff wire, to confirm that the wire has not migrated out of the IVC making a loop in the RA or RV [3, 4]. Furthermore, as dual lumen catheter placement is inherently associated with higher risk for perforation compared to a two-cannula strategy, patients undergoing this procedure should always be prepped and draped from chin to knees so an emergent sternotomy can be performed without delay if perforation occurs [5].

In this patient, the optimal cannulation strategy would be the bicaval approach with two single lumen cannulas performed at bedside using portable image guidance, such as TTE, TEE, or portable X-ray. This is the best means to stabilize a decompensating patient and does not preclude transport to the OR at a later date for fluoroscopic placement of a dual lumen cannula, which enables the patient to sit upright and even to participate in physical therapy.

References

1. Testerman GM, Breitman I, Hensley S. Airway pressure release ventilation in morbidly obese surgical patients with acute lung injury and acute respiratory distress syndrome. Am Surg. 2013;79(3):242–6.
2. Lindholm JA. Cannulation for veno-venous extracorporeal membrane oxygenation. J Thorac Dis. 2018;10(Suppl 5):S606–12.
3. Hemamalini P, Dutta P, Attawar S. Transesophageal echocardiography compared to fluoroscopy for avalon bicaval dual-lumen cannula positioning for venovenous ECMO. Ann Card Anaesth. 2020;23(3):283–7.
4. Hirose H, Yamane K, Marhefka G, Cavarocchi N. Right ventricular rupture and tamponade caused by malposition of the Avalon cannula for venovenous extracorporeal membrane oxygenation. J Cardiothorac Surg. 2012;7:36.
5. Czerwonko ME, Fraga MV, Goldberg DJ, Hedrick HL, Laje P. Cardiovascular perforation during placement of an Avalon Elite(R) Bicaval dual lumen ECMO cannula in a newborn. J Card Surg. 2015;30(4):370–2.

Chapter 43
Reoperative Sternotomy

Brittany Potz and George Tolis

Problem

You have been asked to reoperate on a 72-year-old man 15 years status post mechanical MVR for rheumatic disease, now with severe symptomatic aortic regurgitation. The sternotomy is performed without incident using the oscillating saw, and dissection of the right ventricle and right atrium has been delightfully easy. But the ascending aorta is stubbornly challenging as it is partially rotated toward the right chest. You simply must get some exposure. So, you open the spreader a few more hand cranks and suddenly the upper portion of the sternotomy incision is flooded with a rising tide of dark blood that threatens to sweep you and all you stand for into a hostile and impartial sea. Your heart sinks; it all seemed to be going so well!

Solution

The likely source of the blood is a tear in the innominate vein, which may be tightly adhered to the prior aortic cannulation site underneath and the manubrium above. You kick yourself for failing to re-evaluate the tension on the vein before readjusting the sternal spreader. Recognizing that this thin structure will be intolerant of more tension, you immediately proceed to initiate bypass to decompress the vein

B. Potz
Department of Surgery, Massachusetts General Hospital, Boston, MA, USA
e-mail: bpotz@mgh.harvard.edu

G. Tolis (✉)
Department of Surgery, Brigham and Women's Hospital, Boston, MA, USA
e-mail: gtolis@partners.org

© The Author(s), under exclusive license to Springer Nature Switzerland AG 2022
T. M. Sundt et al. (eds.), *Near Misses in Cardiac Surgery*,
https://doi.org/10.1007/978-3-030-92750-9_43

171

and enable reinfusion of blood. Under more controlled circumstances you repair the tear with a small patch of bovine pericardium knowing that attempts at primary repair will just lead to even more tension and likely an even bigger hole.

Discussion

The incidence of re-entry injury during cardiac surgery is low, only 2–4% [1–3], but this risk increases with each consecutive opening of the sternum [3]. About one third of injuries happen upon re-entry and are associated with a mortality rate up to 25%; however, fully 50% occur during pre-pump dissection [4]. There is remarkable equity among structures, with roughly equal incidence (15%) of innominate vein, right ventricular, aortic, saphenous graft, and ITA injuries. This patient has suffered an avulsion of the innominate vein during—maybe slightly excessive—opening of the chest spreader to improve exposure of the ascending aorta. This is one of many complications that can occur during sternal reentry. An organized approach to sternal reentry can often avoid the creation of these complications. Once they occur, however, they must be dealt with in a systematic way to avoid excessive blood loss prior to repairing the culprit lesion or instituting cardiopulmonary bypass.

A preoperative CT scan should always be obtained prior to sternal reentry as it has been shown to reduce the risk of re-entry injury [2]. It will show the overall rotation of the heart and will define the proximity of the innominate vein, ascending aorta, right ventricle, right atrium, saphenous vein grafts, and IMA grafts to the posterior table of the sternum. The anatomy will direct the surgeon to establish peripheral cardiopulmonary bypass prior to sternal reentry if he or she feels the chest cannot be opened safely. In cases of direct apposition of the ascending aorta (or an aortic pseudoaneurysm) to the sternum, deep hypothermia and circulatory arrest may be the only option for safe reentry. Preoperative CT imaging will also help the surgeon decide if cardiopulmonary bypass should be established prior to attempting the sternotomy to avoid significant blood loss and hemodynamic instability if a venous structure is injured during reentry [5].

If cardiopulmonary bypass has not been established and a tear of the RV, RA or innominate artery occurs, the surgeon needs to quickly decide whether immediate repair is feasible or if cardiopulmonary bypass needs to be established. If an attempt is made to fix the injury site "on the spot," special care needs to be taken to avoid making the problem worse by attempting to expose the bleeding area!

In this scenario, the increased retraction of the sternal edges has resulted in an avulsion of the innominate vein. This can be a challenging injury to address, especially if the avulsion has occurred under the sternum (usually on the left side of the sternum). A left-sided Swan-Ganz catheter further complicates any attempts to repair this injury. Thankfully, the central venous pressure (CVP) is usually low (unless the patient's underlying pathology has led to an increased CVP) and aggressive packing of the neck can temporarily contain the blood loss until cardiopulmonary bypass is established and the injury site is repaired, or the vein is ligated.

Finally, it should be mentioned that obtaining wire access of the femoral artery and vein can significantly decrease the time from injury to institution of cardiopulmonary bypass and should be routinely employed, especially during a surgeon's early career [3]. Additionally, nothing compares with experience when trouble is encountered, so consulting a more senior surgeon is always a good idea [5].

References

1. O'Brien MF, Harrocks S, Clarke A, Garlick B, Barnett AG. How to do safe sternal reentry and the risk factors of redo cardiac surgery: a 21-year review with zero major cardiac injury. J Card Surg. 2002;17(1):4–13. https://doi.org/10.1111/j.1540-8191.2001.tb01213.x. PMID: 12027125.
2. Imran Hamid U, Digney R, Soo L, Leung S, Graham ANJ. Incidence and outcome of re-entry injury in redo cardiac surgery: benefits of preoperative planning, Eur J Cardio-Thorac Surg. 2015;47(5):819–23. https://doi.org/10.1093/ejcts/ezu261.
3. Luciani N, Anselmi A, De Geest R, Martinelli L, Perisano M, Possati G. Extracorporeal circulation by peripheral cannulation before redo stesrnotomy: indications and results, The J Thorac Cardiovasc Surg. 2008;136:572–7. https://doi.org/10.1016/j.jtcvs.2008.02.071.
4. Park CB, Suri RM, Burkhart HM, Greason KL, Dearani JA, Schaff HV, Sundt TM 3rd. Identifying patients at particular risk of injury during repeat sternotomy: analysis of 2555 cardiac reoperations. J Thorac Cardiovasc Surg. 2010;140(5):1028–35. https://doi.org/10.1016/j.jtcvs.2010.07.086 PMID: 20951254.
5. Sabik J, Blackstone E, Houghtaling P, Walts P, Lytle B. Is reoperation still a risk factor in coronary atery bypass surgery? The Ann Thorac Surg. 2005;80:1719–27. https://doi.org/10.1016/j.athoracsur.2005.04.033.

Chapter 44
Sternal Closure: Immediate or Delayed

Greg A. Leya, Arminder S. Jassar, and Kenneth T. Shelton

Problem

It has been a long week already and it is only Tuesday. A late add-on Monday and delays in the OR today between cases have taken their toll. You have just finally drifted off to sleep imagining a well-deserved vacation of sun, sand and tropical refreshments when your resident calls. It's 2:00 AM and a 61 year old patient with a history of prior mechanical aortic valve replacement has just landed in your emergency department as a transfer from an outside hospital where he presented with acute onset of severe chest pain. The chap in the phone does not even need to finish the story—you can see this coming: an acute aortic dissection in a redo chest on coumadin. Rubbing the sleep from your eyes you consider the options. One of your senior colleagues would sit on this one until morning when she and the OR team are fresh figuring that the pericardial adhesions will protect the patient. Unfortunately, you know that there is not a strong evidence base for this approach and the last thing you need is to headline the next Mortality and Morbidity conference. You ask for the patient to be transported to the OR while you make your way to the hospital.

In the operating room the diagnosis is confirmed by transesophageal echo. You peripherally cannulate for bypass and proceed with the operation, encountering significant adhesions and some bleeding after the sternotomy but happily without entering the aorta. It is not an easy operation—graft replacement of the root and

G. A. Leya · A. S. Jassar
Department of Surgery, Massachusetts General Hospital, Boston, MA, USA
e-mail: gleya@mgh.harvard.edu

A. S. Jassar
e-mail: ajassar@mgh.harvard.edu

K. T. Shelton (✉)
Department of Anesthesia, Massachusetts General Hospital, Boston, MA, USA
e-mail: kshelton@mgh.harvard.edu

© The Author(s), under exclusive license to Springer Nature Switzerland AG 2022   175
T. M. Sundt et al. (eds.), *Near Misses in Cardiac Surgery*,
https://doi.org/10.1007/978-3-030-92750-9_44

ascending aorta sewing to the cuff of a mechanical prosthesis, reimplanting the coronaries proximally and distally a 2/3 arch. The right coronary was dissected so you took extra care to carefully reconstruct the button. When the clamp comes off a normal rhythm returns much to your relief. Are we out of the woods? Amazingly after prolonged bypass and clamp times you are able to wean the patient off bypass and close the sternum. As you pull the wires together and ask the circulating nurse to turn on your favorite George Straight music station, the anesthesiologist complains that they are unhappy with the right ventricular function. Resisting the urge to complain that they are never happy with the right ventricular function you look up to see that the CVP is now 18 mmHg and the systemic pressure has fallen; tamponade physiology. You relax the wires and the CVP drops while the systemic pressure rises. You have to admit, the heart looks boggy and edematous. You know the bleeding will be less if you can oppose the sternal edges. Bleeding or hemodynamic deterioration? You are between Scylla and Charybdis. When will this operation will be over?

Solution

Discretion being the better part of valor, you decide to leave the chest open to allow for cardiac decompression. You modify a 60-cc syringe at both ends, wedge it between the two halves of the sternum, and overlay an Esmark with Ioban dressing. You then take the patient back to the ICU.

The patient is maintained on the ventilator and his vasopressor and inotrope requirements improve. You return to the operating room on post-operative day 2 for mediastinal washout. The surgical sites are hemostatic, and you are able to definitively close the sternum.

Discussion

First described in the 1970s, delayed sternal closure is performed in approximately 1–4% of cardiac cases. It is particularly common in the pediatric population, with numerous case series describing the merits of delayed sternal closure in congenital operations. An open chest allows for decompression of the mediastinal structures and for easy accessibility in the setting of massive bleeding or difficult hemostasis. As such, the primary indications for delayed sternal closure at the end of a cardiac case include mechanical restriction of cardiac diastolic function manifest as hemodynamic instability or cardiac arrythmias, in addition to myocardial edema, RV failure, intractable bleeding, or elevated ventilator pressures and poor lung compliance in the setting of sternal closure.

The above case presents a patient with many of the risk factors for delayed sternal closure, including re-operation, prolonged cardiopulmonary bypass and cross clamp times, and need for blood product resuscitation. In this case, the patient was able to have definitive sternal closure on his first takeback to the OR, whereas it is even more common for patients to require one or more mediastinal washouts prior to definitive closure. Whereas this patient was dressed with a simple dressing of Esmark and Ioban, vacuum-assisted closure devices have gained popularity among surgeons as they may prevent the catastrophic complication of a right ventricular tear occurring with coughing ("the big red scream").

While in the ICU, patients with open chest wounds are kept intubated under sedation. While waking trials are appropriate to assess neurologic function, one can expect that the patient will need full ventilator support. Generating enough negative intrathoracic pressure to maintain adequate minute ventilation is difficult with pressure support settings even with advanced ICU ventilators in patients with open chests. Hemostasis is monitored using chest tubes and hemodynamic parameters. Mediastinal infection remains a primary concern for many ICU providers but complicates only 1–4% of delayed sternal closures. While definitive evidence for or against antibiotic prophylaxis is lacking and there are no definitive guidelines, most providers are pulling away from empiric broad spectrum antibiotics as we become better stewards of antibiotic use, although the choice of antibiotic and duration remains highly variable.

Bibliography

1. Adsumelli RS, Shapiro JR, Shah PM, Martella AT, Afifi AY, Risher WB, Hicks GL. Hemodynamic effects of chest closure in adult patients undergoing cardiac surgery. J Cardiothorac Vasc Anesth. 2001;15(5):589–92.
2. Furnary AP, Magovern JA, Simpson KA, Magovern JG. Prolonged open sternotomy and delayed sternal closure after cardiac operations. Ann Thorac Surg. 1992;54:233–9.
3. Gielchinsky I, Parsonnet V, Krishnan B, Silidker M, Abel RM. Delayed sternal closure following open-heart operation. Ann Thorac Surg. 1981;32:273–7.
4. Anderson CA, Filsoufi F, Aklog L, Farivar RS, Byrne JG, Adams DH. Liberal use of delayed sternal closure for postcardiotomy hemodynamic instability. Ann Thorac Surg. 2002;73:1484–8.
5. Estrera AL, Porat EE, Miller CM 3rd, Meada R, Achouh PE, Irani AD, Safi HJ. Outcomes of delayed sternal closure after complex aortic surgery. Eur J CTS. 2008;33:1039–42.
6. Elassal AA, Eldib OS, Dohain AM, Abdelmohsen GA, Abdalla AH, Al-Radi OO. Delayed sternal closure in congenital heart surgery: a risk-benefit analysis. The Hear Surg Forum. 2019; 22(5).
7. Christenson JT, Maurice J, Simonet F, Velebit V, Schmuziger M. Open chest and delayed sternal closure after cardiac surgery. Eur J CTS. 1996;10:305–11.
8. Boeken U, Feindt P, Schurr P, Assmann A, Akhyari P, Lichtenberg A. Delayed sternal closure after cardiac surgery. J Card Surg. 2011;26:22–7.
9. Eckardt JL, Wanek MR, Udeh CI, Neuner EA, Fraser TG, Attia T, Roselli EE. Evaluation of prophylactic antibiotic use for delayed sternal closure after cardiothoracic operation. Ann Thorac Surg. 2018;105:1365–9.

Chapter 45
Suction Event After LVAD Placement

S. Alireza Rabi and David A. D'Alessandro

Problem

It's a warm day in July and the streets of Boston are buzzing with activity. You have a short day in the clinic and afterward you go for a stroll along Charles Street. The plan for the afternoon is to place a left ventricular assist device (LVAD) for Mr. C, a 68-year-old retired teacher with ischemic cardiomyopathy. At the age of 62 he had a coronary stent placed for myocardial ischemia. Since then, he has been followed by the Heart Failure team. Despite aggressive medical therapy he has developed worsening heart function. He is also being evaluated for heart transplantation and has no contraindications. However, because of his progressive symptoms and concerning renal dysfunction, the plan is to proceed with LVAD implantation as a bridge-to-transplant.

At the beginning of the case, the right atrial pressure is 15 mmHg with PA systolic and diastolic values of 25 and 12 mmHg, respectively. Concerned about these numbers, you decide to proceed with the planned operation anyway. After a technically uncomplicated procedure you are satisfied with the location of the cannulae as the perfusionist starts the device and quickly ramps up to full speed. Initially, the flows are satisfactory, and the mean arterial pressure remains in the low to mid-60 s with minimal inotropic and vasopressor support. Hemostasis looks good and you have just started to close when the device alarms because of a series of suction events. The central venous pressure is elevated. The transesophageal echocardiogram confirms that the placement of the inflow cannula is appropriate; however, the interventricular septum is now shifted towards the left ventricle.

S. A. Rabi · D. A. D'Alessandro (✉)
Department of Surgery, Massachusetts General Hospital, Boston, MA, USA
e-mail: dadalessandro@mgh.harvard.edu

S. A. Rabi
e-mail: srabi@mgh.harvard.edu

© The Author(s), under exclusive license to Springer Nature Switzerland AG 2022
T. M. Sundt et al. (eds.), *Near Misses in Cardiac Surgery*,
https://doi.org/10.1007/978-3-030-92750-9_45

179

Solution

Recognizing the underlying problem as RV failure, you quickly turn the LVAD flows down, ask the anesthesiologist to initiate vasopressors to keep the mean arterial pressure (MAP) greater than 70, and to administer milrinone, moderate-dose epinephrine, and inhaled epoprostenol. You also ask him to show you the four-chamber view of the heart to better monitor the impact of your interventions on the right heart. After several minutes, the right atrial pressures start to decrease, and the PA pulsatility index (PAPi) increases above 2. Once you are satisfied that the RV has somewhat recovered its function, you ask the perfusionist to gradually increase the LVAD flow while keeping an eye on the four-chamber view of the heart. You aim to set the LVAD flow at a rate that causes slight bowing of the interventricular septum towards the RV. Once you achieve this, you ask the perfusionist to maintain that speed. You are happy to see that the PA pressures remain stable and the echocardiogram shows adequate RV function. You are fully aware that if the above maneuvers had not successfully rescued the RV function, unplanned biventricular assistance (BiVAD) might have become necessary. Over the next 48 h you plan to increase the LVAD flows gradually.

Discussion

A "suction event" is a dynamic process whereby the wall of the LV collapses and obstructs the inflow cannula of the LVAD device. The major causes of a suction event are insufficient preload, RV failure, inappropriate angulation of the inflow cannula during the implantation, and arrhythmias. In this case, the high CVP and echocardiographic images rule out low volume and inappropriate cannula position as potential causes. On the other hand, concerningly low preoperative PA pressures, in addition to the echocardiographic finding of septal bowing towards the LV, point to right heart failure as the cause. The low systemic pressures will cause an increase in LVAD flow as centrifugal pumps are afterload sensistive. Rapid LV decompression can shift the ventricular septum towards the left which further compromises the baseline RV dysfunction. Treatment included initiating inotropic support for the RV which was ianappropriated underutilized initially, administration of a pulmonary vasodilator and a reduction in pump speed with afterload augmentation to prevent a recurrent event.

Several parameters have been developed to predict RV failure after LV placement. The PA pulsatility index (PAPi) calculated as: [(pulmonary artery systolic pressure—pulmonary artery diastolic pressure)/right atrial pressure] has gained popularity. Values less than 2 are predictive of RV failure after LVAD implantation.

Bibliography

1. Meineri M, Van Rensburg AE, Vegas A. Right ventricular failure after LVAD implantation: prevention and treatment. Best Pract Res Clin Anaesthesiol. 2012;26(2):217–29. https://doi.org/10.1016/j.bpa.2012.03.006.
2. Kochav SM, Flores RJ, Truby LK, Topkara VK. Prognostic impact of pulmonary artery pulsatility index (PAPi) in patients with advanced heart failure: insights from the ESCAPE trial. J Card Fail. 2018;24(7):453–9. https://doi.org/10.1016/j.cardfail.2018.03.008.
3. Kang G, Ha R, Banerjee D. Pulmonary artery pulsatility index predicts right ventricular failure after left ventricular assist device implantation. J Heart Lung Transplant. 2016;35(1):67–73. https://doi.org/10.1016/j.healun.2015.06.009.
4. Reesink K, Dekker A, Nagel TV, Beghi C, Leonardi F, Botti P, De Cicco G, Lorusso R, Veen F, Maessen J. Suction due to left ventricular assist: implications for device control and management. J Artif Organs. 2007;31(7):542–9. https://doi.org/10.1111/j.1525-1594.2007.00420.x.
5. Guglin M, Zucker MJ, Borlaug BA, Breen E, Cleveland J, Johnson MR, Panjrath GS, Patel JK, Starling RC, Bozkurt B. ACC heart failur and transplant member section and leadership council. Evaluation for heart transplantation and LVAD implantation: JACC council perspectives. JACC. 2020;75(12):1471–87. https://doi.org/10.1016/j.jacc.2020.01.034.

Chapter 46
Thrombosed Mechanical Valve

Antonia Kreso and Serguei Melnitchouk

Problem

The emergency department at your hospital is the busiest in the city, with an eclectic blend of high-end complex patients from all over the region to the local clientele typical of any urban center. While the former present challenging diagnostic dilemmas, in many ways so do the latter. Today you have been asked by the emergency department to see a 58-year-old male who recently had mitral valve surgery elsewhere. The emergency department physician tells you the patient has a history of excessive alcohol use, falls, and epilepsy for which he is taking carbamazepine. From the records, it appears the patient had a mitral valve replacement with a mechanical valve for mitral insufficiency caused by endocarditis 3 months previously. He was discharged on warfarin therapy but has poor social support and was lost to follow-up. He now presents with shortness of breath.

You examine the patient and notice he is in volume overload with a blood pressure of 110/60 mmHg. His extremities are warm. You hear bilateral rales and muffled closing clicks. You check the patient's labs and your suspected diagnosis is supported when you see an INR of 1.3. The emergency room doctor informs you the patient's preliminary echocardiogram showed a new gradient across the mitral valve and a mitral valve area of 0.9 cm^2.

A. Kreso · S. Melnitchouk (✉)
Department of Surgery, Massachusetts General Hospital, Boston, MA, USA
e-mail: smelnitchouk@mgh.harvard.edu

A. Kreso
e-mail: akreso@mgh.harvard.edu

© The Author(s), under exclusive license to Springer Nature Switzerland AG 2022
T. M. Sundt et al. (eds.), *Near Misses in Cardiac Surgery*,
https://doi.org/10.1007/978-3-030-92750-9_46

Solution

You review the echocardiogram images, which do not clearly demonstrate motion of two leaflets. You then order a quick fluoroscopy exam, and your suspicion is confirmed—the RAO cranial projection demonstrates that one leaflet of the mitral valve prosthesis is not moving, while the other one has completely normal motion. You start the patient on a heparin infusion and admit him to the intensive care unit for close monitoring. You discuss further options with the patient. Although it is a left-sided valve, because there does not appear to be a large thrombus burden, the risk of thromboembolism is relatively low. The risks of intracranial hemorrhage associated with fibrinolysis are not insignificant, but re-operation carries substantial risk. The following morning the leaflet still appears stuck by transthoracic echocardiogram, so you begin a slow infusion of fibrinolytic therapy. Repeat fluoroscopy exam confirms that both leaflets are now opening freely, and a transthoracic echocardiogram confirms an improved gradient across the mitral valve prosthesis. The patient does not have any neurological consequences and recovers after fibrinolytic therapy, avoiding surgical intervention. You recommend transitioning to Coumadin with a target INR of 3–4. You wish the patient had received a bioprosthesis, but it appears you and he have dodged a bullet—for now.

Discussion

Acute mechanical prosthetic valve thrombosis requires urgent diagnosis, evaluation, and therapy as rapid deterioration can occur. Obstruction of mechanical prosthetic heart valves may be caused by thrombus formation, new infective endocarditis, or pannus ingrowth. Further diagnostic workup may include multimodal imaging in the form of CT scan, transthoracic/transesophageal echocardiogram, or fluoroscopy. Fluoroscopy is a useful adjunct to help diagnose a stuck leaflet. Using the tilting disk projection with X-ray beams parallel to both the valve ring plane and the tilting axis of the disks (usually RAO cranial projection), opening/closing angles of the disks of the valve can be obtained and serially tracked following therapy.

Thrombolytic therapy is an acceptable approach to prosthetic valve thrombosis among patients with recent onset thrombosis, mild (NYHA class I or II symptoms) and less than 0.8 cm^2 thrombus burden. A trial of IV heparin for 48 h is reasonable and sometimes successful. However, if full anticoagulation with heparin is not successful, it should be followed either with fibrinolysis or surgical intervention. Patients with a large thrombus burden or a mobile thrombus greater than 0.8 cm^2 are at higher risk of stroke from embolic phenomena. Patients with a history of hemorrhagic stroke, recent trauma or internal bleeding, as well as those patients with severe systemic hypertension, are at increased risk of complications related to fibrinolytic therapy [1, 2].

Slow-infusion fibrinolytic therapy has higher success rates and lower complication rates than prior high-dose regimens and is effective in patients previously thought to require urgent surgical intervention. For example, slow-infusion low-dose fibrinolytic protocols have shown success rates >90%, with embolic event rates <2% and major bleeding rates <2% [3]. Factors that have been proposed as a guide to favor surgery include readily available surgical expertise, low surgical risk, contra-indication to fibrinolysis, recurrent valve thrombosis, NYHA class IV, large clot (>0.8 cm^2), left atrial thrombus, concomitant coronary artery disease in need of revascularization, other valve disease, possible pannus, and patient choice [4].

If thrombolysis is contraindicated, emergency reoperation is necessary. At surgery, the valve can be inspected for presence of pannus impinging upon leaflet motion and predisposing to thrombosis. If the valve leaflet can be liberated easily and the thrombus burden is small with no pannus apparent, the valve can simply be cleaned and, if necessary, rotated. Not infrequently, however, thrombus burden is significant, and it is more straightforward to simply remove the old valve. The decision about placing another mechanical valve versus replacing it with a tissue valve needs to be individualized in the context of each patient. Patient age and comorbidities need to be identified, along with the patient's valve preference after risks and benefits of a mechanical versus bioprosthetic valve are considered. Consideration of future valve-in-valve options exist for older patients whose anatomy allows placement of a larger sized valve. Finally, counselling patients on medications and adherence to INR checks is instrumental in achieving long-term durable results. This is especially true in high-risk populations where it may be difficult for patients to access care or have close follow-up of INRs.

Bibliography

1. Nishimura RA, Otto CM, Bonow RO, Carabello BA, Erwin JP 3rd, Guyton RA, O'Gara PT, Ruiz CE, Skubas NJ, Sorajja P, Sundt TM 3rd, Thomas JD, AHA/ACA Task Force members. 2014 AHA/ACC guideline for the management of patients with valvular heart disease: executive summary. Circulation. 2014;129:2440–92.
2. Nishimura RA, Otto CM, Bonow RO, Carabello BA, Erwin JP 3rd, Fleisher LA, Jneid H, Mack MJ, McLeod CJ, O'Gara PT, Rigolin VH, Sundt TM 3rd, Thompson A. AHA/ACC focused update of the 2014 AHA/ACC guidelines for the management of patients with valvular heart disease. JACC. 2017;70(2):252–89.
3. Özkan M, Cakal B, Karakoyun S, Gursoy OM, Cevik C, Kalcik M, Oguz AE, Gunduz S, Astarcioglu MA, Aykan AC, Bayram Z, Biteker M, Kaynak E, Kahveci G, Duran NE, Yildiz M. Thrombolytic therapy for the treatment of prosthetic heart valve thrombosis in pregnancy with low-dose, slow infusion of tissue-type plasminogen activator. Circulation. 2013;128:532–40.
4. Özkan M, Gunduz S, Gursoy OM, Karakoyun S, Astarcioglu MA, Kalcik M, Aykan AC, Cakal B, Byram Z, Oguz AE, Erturk E, Yesin M, KalikGokdeniz T, Duran NE, Yildiz M, Esen AM. Ultraslow thrombolytic therapy: a novel strategy in the management of prosthetic mechanical valve Thrombosis and the predictors of outcome: the Ultra-slow PROMETEE trial. Am Heart J. 2015;170:409–18.

Chapter 47
Valve-sparing Aortic Root Repair

Andrew A. C. Baldwin, William Shi, and Thoralf M. Sundt

Problem

You have just removed the cross-clamp after performing a valve-sparing aortic root replacement (reimplantation technique) in a 55-year-old athlete who presented with an aortic root aneurysm and adamant he did not want to take Coumadin. You trained under a leader in the field, and your new partners were excited to recruit you to be the only surgeon in the region proficient in valve-sparing techniques. Several other surgeons in the department have come into your operating room to marvel at this technical achievement. The transesophageal echocardiogram demonstrates no aortic regurgitation. You are certain once word spreads amongst the referring cardiologists that your practice as a complex aortic surgeon will grow exponentially.

You wean from bypass uneventfully. Prior to administering protamine, you notice some bright red blood pooling posterior to the aortic root. You manipulate the graft and suction around the area as best you can but cannot identify the source of bleeding. Fearing a problem with the left coronary button, you resume full bypass and carefully inspect the graft. The coronary anastomosis looks perfect. Reassured, but a bit puzzled, you wean from bypass a second time only to see the pericardial cavity again fill with bright red blood. You don't remember seeing this problem during your fellowship experience, and you wonder what needs to be fixed—and how.

A. A. C. Baldwin
Division of Cardiac Surgery, Straub Medical Center, Honolulu, HI, USA
e-mail: Andrew.Baldwin@hphmg.org

W. Shi
Department of Surgery, Massachusetts General Hospital, Boston, MA, USA
e-mail: WYSGI@mgh.harvard.edu

T. M. Sundt (✉)
Division of Cardiac Surgery, Massachusetts General Hospital, Boston, MA, USA
e-mail: tsundt@mgh.harvard.edu

© The Author(s), under exclusive license to Springer Nature Switzerland AG 2022
T. M. Sundt et al. (eds.), *Near Misses in Cardiac Surgery*,
https://doi.org/10.1007/978-3-030-92750-9_47

You look around meticulously but you are unable to find an obvious focus. You are frustrated by the blood running down from the needle-holes in the graft material and by the beads of sweat gathering at your neck and running down your back. All eyes are upon you! The anaesthesiologists and operating room nurses begin to suspect something is wrong, and you can hear murmurs from around the room "why didn't we do it the way we always do it? We should have just done a good old fashioned composite root replacement."

Solution

Given the bright red appearance of the blood, you surmise that the source must be left-sided: either the aorta, the left ventricle, or the left atrium. Since it resolves with resumption of cardiopulmonary bypass, you reason that the bleeding must not be aortic despite your initial concern about the left coronary button. After all, when you gave antegrade cardioplegia down the graft after completion of the valve and coronary button re-implantation, the suture lines were all hemostatic.

You instruct the anaesthesiologist to administer protamine, and pack the area with gauze, hoping it will stop. You spend the next 15 min inserting drains and ensuring hemostasis of the sternum and anterior mediastinum. The anaesthesiologist informs you that all the protamine has been administered and that the ACT is back to baseline. Given the long bypass run, the team also performed a thromboelastogram which shows essentially normal clotting function.

With apprehension, you remove the gauzes and note that although the hemostasis is generally excellent, you still see bright red blood slowly pooling behind the aorta, albeit much slower than before. You retract the aorta to the left and finally, without blood running down from above since the suture holes are now hemostatic, you spot the culprit.

There is a focus of bleeding coming from a small injury in the roof of the left atrium, along with several smaller bleeders from the surrounding epicardium you had dissected so you could reach the subannular plane. You ask your assistant to retract the aorta leftward, and using a 5/0 polypropylene suture, you oversew the left atrial roof and cauterize the epicardial bleeders. You pack the area with gauze again, and after five minutes, return to find that the gauzes are completely dry. There is no more pooling of blood.

Exhausted both physically and emotionally, you ask your assistant to close. You scrub out and check your phone to find three new referrals for root aneurysms.

Discussion

Bleeding after aortic root replacement is problematic owing to the difficulty of visualizing the suture lines, especially the proximal ones. With multiple suture lines in graft material, needle hole bleeding can seem torrential, but will in fact stop with protamine. Placing repair stiches in this area is also technically challenging, and can at times, exacerbate the problem if performed without good visualization. It can be difficult to know whether it is appropriate to stay on bypass and manipulate the graft, to continue to search for points of bleeding, or to come off and administer protamine hoping for the best.

These operations require a certain degree of mobilization of tissue around the aorta and aortic root. For a composite root replacement, this can be kept to a relative minimum; however, the surgeon must nonetheless mobilize the coronary buttons, as well as any connective tissue or adhesions between the aorta and surrounding structures, namely, the pulmonary artery, the left atrium, the right atrium, and right ventricle. For a valve-sparing root replacement, a more extensive dissection must be carried out around the aortic root to the subannular plane to enable the valve to be reimplanted inside a Dacron graft [1]. In patients with large aneurysms, acute or chronic dissections, as well as reoperations, circumferential mobilization of the aorta can be difficult and injury to adjacent structures may not be easily recognized. As well, the subannular sutures in a valve-sparing operation can cause subtle tears in the roof of the left atrium as it is particularly thin adjacent to the aortic root proximal to Bachmann's Bundle, especially in patients with poor tissue quality.

In this case, however, the bleeding is left-sided. Most often the culprit in this scenario is the left coronary button or distal aortic anastomosis, but these sources should be apparent as soon as the clamp comes off and the root is pressurized. In this case, it was only when you withdrew from bypass that the bleeding revealed itself. The source, then, must either be the left ventricle or left atrium. If the former, it is more likely that a jet of blood will be identified, even if perhaps a bit less accessible for repair.

In this case, the bleeding was noted only once off bypass, when the heart was filled under physiological pressures, leading to bright red bleeding from the left atrial roof. However, once back on bypass, with the left heart empty and the left atrial pressure being essentially zero, no bleeding could be appreciated. This same phenomenon may be observed after heart transplantation if the left atrial suture line is not perfectly tight.

The presence of dark red bleeding originating anteriorly from the root once off bypass may suggest bleeding from dissection of the right atrium or right ventricular muscle. Slow bleeding from this area is not uncommon, and generally resolves with administration of protamine, reversal of any coagulopathy, and gentle packing of the areas with gauze. Topical sealants may also be beneficial [2]. Also, it is useful to briefly fill the heart once all the dissection is done, prior to commencing any reconstruction, as any injury to the RVOT, PA or, the left atrium is readily visible and straightforward to repair without the aortic root or coronary arteries in the way.

Brisk bleeding of bright blood that rapidly pools immediately after cross-clamp release suggests an arterial source, such as that of the coronary buttons or the proximal anastomosis. If this cannot be addressed with the heart beating, then it may require a period of re-cross clamping to adequately expose and visualize the source before repair sutures can be placed accurately and safely.

It is worth recalling that in a composite root replacement, bleeding emanating from underneath the sewing ring of the valve prosthesis may result if the prosthesis has not been seated satisfactorily. This bleeding will usually be substantial and be readily identifiable, even if less accessible for repair. This situation would result in a paravalvular leak in a standard aortic valve replacement. However, in a composite root replacement, any defect here results in bleeding from the ventricle into the pericardial space—which obviously has potentially catastrophic consequences. If this occurs, additional sutures can sometimes be placed from outside the aorta into the sewing ring. On occasion, it may be necessary to re-arrest the heart, take down the distal anastomosis and reinforce the proximal anastomosis either with a running suture or with additional pledgeted sutures. It may even be necessary to take down the coronary buttons to get access. A leak such as this is less likely after a reimplantation as the running suture to reimplant the valve is usually quite hemostatic.

In rare instances, if the bleeding seems otherwise uncontrollable, a Cabrol baffle [3] can be created, covering the root with a pericardial patch sewn to the pulmonary artery (left), superior vena cava (right), innominate vein (superiorly) and right ventricle (inferiorly), with a stab wound into the innominate vein or right atrium for decompression. This requires that the transverse sinus be closed either thanks to adhesions in a redo setting or with an additional patch. While this is not an ideal solution, it may get the patient out of the operating room alive, and the fistulas typically close on their own due to the low-pressure system.

As mentioned in this case, to reduce the likelihood of having bleeding in inaccessible locations, pressurizing proximal suture lines upon their completion with antegrade cardioplegia enables their repair before completion of the distal aortic anastomosis, which renders visualization and access more difficult [4].

Understanding the potential pitfalls of each step of an aortic root replacement is essential to minimizing operative hazards and complications.

References

1. Cameron D, Vricella L. Valve-sparing aortic root replacement with the Valsalva Graft. Op Tech Thorac Cardiovasc Surg. 2009;14:297–308.
2. Bracey A, Shander A, Aronson S, Boucher BA, Calcaterra D, Chu MWA, Culbertson R, Jabr K, Kehlet H, Lattouf O, Malaisrie SC, Mazer CD, Oberhoffer MM, Ozawa S, Price T, Rosengart T, Spiess BD, Turchetti G. The use of topical hemostatic agents in cardiothoracic surgery. Ann Thorac Surg. 2017;104:353–60.
3. Cabrol C, Gandjbakhch, Cham B. Anverismes de l'aorte ascendante. Remplacement total avec des arteres coronaires. Nouv Presse Med. 1978;7:363–5.
4. Bayfield MS, Kron IL. Reducing bleeding after replacement of the aortic root. Ann Thorac Surg. 1995;60:1130–1.

Chapter 48
Acute Aortic Dissection

Rizwan Q. Attia and Arminder S. Jassar

Problem

You are contacted by the resident on call who reports that a 45-year-old hypertensive man has just presented in the ER with severe central chest pain radiating to the back and with "pins and needles" in his left leg. Upon evaluation in the ED, he appears anxious and reports ongoing severe chest pain. He is hypertensive with a BP of 180/110 mmHg and in sinus tachycardia with a rate of 100 bpm. Labetalol infusion is begun, and he is whisked off to CT scan where an IV contrast CTA reveals a diagnosis of a Stanford Type A/De Bakey type I aortic dissection. The dissection flap extends from the aortic root to the iliac arteries. The true lumen supplies all end-organ beds except the SMA and left iliac which come off the false lumen. You decide to take the patient to the operating room for emergent repair of his aortic dissection. After a long case, you manage to preserve the aortic valve and replace the ascending aorta and hemiarch with a Dacron prosthesis under deep hypothermic circulatory arrest. You are pleased when the patient comes off cardiopulmonary bypass easily with good LV function and minimal aortic regurgitation on TEE. Even the bleeding does not seem that bad and you begin to think you might make your dinner engagement after all. Confidant that the gods are smiling on you, you discuss giving protamine. However, the anesthetist informs you that the patient has remained acidotic since coming off bypass. The pulse is 86 with DDD pacing, BP 110/60 mmHg on 1 mcg/kg/min norepinephrine, 0.5mcg/kg/min

R. Q. Attia
National Health Service, London, UK
e-mail: rizwanattia@icloud.com

A. S. Jassar (✉)
Department of Surgery, Massachusetts General Hospital, Boston, MA, USA
e-mail: ajasser@mgh.harvard.edu

© The Author(s), under exclusive license to Springer Nature Switzerland AG 2022   191
T. M. Sundt et al. (eds.), *Near Misses in Cardiac Surgery*,
https://doi.org/10.1007/978-3-030-92750-9_48

epinephrine with a rising lactate at 10 mmol/L. You surmise that the acidosis is a lingering effect of the dissection and will soon begin to resolve once the patient is resuscitated in the ICU. You head off to dictate the operative note. Upon removing the surgical drapes, the resident notices that the patient's left leg is pale and cooler than the right leg. She is unable to get pedal doppler signals.

Solution

You ask your anesthesiologist to interrogate the descending thoracic aorta on TEE to assess the dissection flap. As best as can be seen, the true lumen appears to be reasonably well expanded in the proximal descending aorta. You decide the patient requires a repeat imaging study either with CTA, conventional angiography, or intravascular ultrasound to determine the dissection flap dynamics and branch vessel reperfusion. You request the vascular surgery team to come to the operating room to assess the patient and they share your concerns about the possibility of ongoing malperfusion. The patient is transferred safely to the adjacent hybrid suite where angiography confirms occlusion of the left iliac artery and reduced flow in the SMA. The vascular surgery team places an endovascular stent from the true lumen of the aorta into the SMA as well as a second stent in the left common iliac artery. Repeat angiography demonstrates restoration of SMA and left iliac blood flow, and now there is a palpable left femoral pulse. Owing to the long period of malperfusion, you are concerned about reperfusion injury. Therefore, a prophylactic fasciotomy of the left leg is performed. An exploratory laparotomy reveals that the bowel remains viable. The patient is transferred in stable but critical condition to the ICU where his clinical state improves gradually over the next 24 h.

Discussion

Mortality and morbidity are much higher in patients who have malperfusion at presentation with aortic dissection [1, 2]. End-organ malperfusion affects up to 30% of patients and increases the mortality rate to 40–50% [3, 4]. Distal malperfusion is related to large re-entry tears and true lumen collapse in the descending aorta causing impairment of the abdominal visceral, renal, and peripheral circulations. Central aortic repair with resection of the proximal entry tear and redirection of flow into the true lumen will resolve the distal malperfusion in most but not all cases [5, 6]. With dynamic malperfusion, the true lumen may remain compressed due to false lumen pressurization resulting in occlusion of the branch vessel orifice by the dissection flap. Static malperfusion occurs when the intimal flap extends into the branch vessels, with subsequent thrombosis of the false lumen and occlusion of the true lumen. In many cases, a combination of both static and dynamic components may be present. When there is a concern about ongoing malperfusion after central aortic repair, prompt evaluation and treatment are of paramount importance.

In this patient, the absent leg pulse after ascending aortic replacement provided an early warning sign on physical exam. Mesenteric malperfusion, however, is hard to evaluate, and may only be recognized late during ICU care, by which time irreversible visceral ischemia may have occurred. A high index of suspicion must be maintained in patients with radiologic features of end-organ malperfusion. Patients with clinical or metabolic signs of malperfusion at the end of surgical repair or in the ICU require further imaging investigation. Either repeat contrast CT imaging or invasive evaluation with angiography or IVUS plays an important role in diagnosis. While central aortic repair may relieve dynamic obstruction, once end-organ damage has occurred or branch vessel thrombosis is present due to static occlusion, malperfusion is not reliably resolved by proximal aortic repair alone. Treatment may involve endovascular treatment with stent graft placement in the descending aorta to re-expand the true lumen, fenestration of the dissection membrane, or stenting of the target branch vessel to restore flow. Additional procedures such as bowel resection or leg fasciotomies may be necessary based on the duration and severity of the malperfusion. A multi-disciplinary team approach is the best way to provide patient care as vascular, general surgery, and intensive care team input is needed.

Controversy remains about the optimal initial management of patients presenting with malperfusion and end organ dysfunction. Given the poor outcomes reported in this setting with primary central aortic repair in the hope of restoring flow to the compromised beds, some centers advocate initial reperfusion of the malperfused organ prior to central repair [3, 7], either with endovascular fenestration of the dissection membrane or with stent graft deployment in the descending aorta for true lumen expansion. The patient is then monitored carefully in the ICU and brought back to the operating room for definitive repair once the malperfusion resolves. This delayed operative strategy, however, can result in interval aortic rupture, cardiac tamponade, and even death due to the complications of malperfusion. Others have advocated for an aggressive approach to central aortic repair, including total arch replacement with frozen elephant trunk or hemiarch replacement plus antegrade thoracic endovascular aortic repair (TEVAR) of the descending thoracic aorta for DeBakey I dissection with distal malperfusion [8, 9]. Others have adopted a strategy of 'verified complete reperfusion' for all DeBakey type I dissections [10]. This involves an early discussion between the cardiac and vascular surgery teams regarding the operative plan, and utilization of the hybrid operating room for all patients with aortic dissection. After central aortic repair, distal true lumen expansion and reestablishment of visceral perfusion is confirmed using TEE, IVUS, or angiography. In case of ongoing compromise, additional interventions are performed immediately, before leaving the operating room. This approach allows for complete resolution of distal malperfusion while avoiding the complications associated with the delayed central aortic repair.

References

1. Kawahito K, Kimura N, Yamaguchi A, Aizawa K. Malperfusion in type A aortic dissection: results of emergency central aortic repair. Gen Thorac Cardiovasc Surg. 2019;67(7):594–601.
2. Vallabhajosyula P, Gottret JP, Menon R, et al. Central repair with antegrade TEVAR for Malperfusion syndromes in acute DeBakey I aortic dissection. Ann Thorac Surg. 2017;103 (3):748–55.
3. Yang B, Norton EL, Rosati CM, et al. Managing patients with acute type A aortic dissection and mesenteric malperfusion syndrome: a 20-year experience. J Thorac Cardiovasc Surg. 2019;158(3):675-687.e4.
4. Di Eusanio M, Trimarchi S, Patel HJ, et al. Clinical presentation, management, and short-term outcome of patients with type A acute dissection complicated by mesenteric malperfusion: observations from the international registry of acute aortic dissection. J Thorac Cardiovasc Surg. 2013;145(2):385-390.e1.
5. Easo J, Weigang E, Hölzl PPF, et al. Influence of operative strategy for the aortic arch in DeBakey type I aortic dissection: analysis of the German registry for acute aortic dissection type A. J Thorac Cardiovasc Surg. 2012;144(3):617–23.
6. Berretta P, Trimarchi S, Patel HJ, Gleason TG, Eagle KA, Di Eusanio M. Malperfusion syndromes in type A aortic dissection: what we have learned from IRAD. J Vis Surg. 2018;4 (3):65–75.
7. Yang B, Patel HJ, Williams DM, Dasika NL, Deeb GM. Management of type A dissection with malperfusion. Ann Cardiothorac Surg. 2016;5(4):265–74.
8. Attia RQ, Cameron DE, Sundt TM III, Jassar AS. Total arch replacement in the treatment of acute type A aortic dissection. J Vis Surg. 2020. https://doi.org/10.21037/jovs-20-125.
9. Czerny M, Schmidli J, Bertoglio L, et al. Clinical cases referring to diagnosis and management of patients with thoracic aortic pathologies involving the aortic arch: a companion document of the 2018 European association for cardio-thoracic surgery (EACTS) and the European society for vascular surgery (ESVS) expert consensus document addressing current options and recommendations for the treatment of thoracic aortic pathologies involving the aortic arch. Eur J Vasc Endovasc Surg. 2019;57(3):452–60.
10. Axtell A, Eagleton M, Conrad M, Isselbacher E, Sundt T, Jassar A. Total arch replacement and frozen elephant trunk for acute complicated type B dissection. Ann Thorac Surg. 2020;110(3):e213–6.

Chapter 49
Hypotension on Bypass

Myles E. Lee and Thoralf M. Sundt

Problem

A 60-year-old patient with progressive angina is found to have triple-vessel disease
in need of coronary bypass grafting. Your colleague who normally operates at the
satellite center of your practice is on vacation, so you decide to help her out and do
the case. In the operating room, the patient maintains normal hemodynamics during
a smooth anesthetic induction, endotracheal intubation, prepping, draping, and
sternotomy. You perform routine cannulations of the ascending aorta, insert a
two-stage venous drainage cannula into the right atrium and the inferior vena cava,
and a catheter into the ascending aorta to serve as an aortic root vent and as a
conduit for the administration of antegrade cardioplegia. You begin cardiopulmonary bypass and prepare to put the finishing touches on the internal thoracic
artery pedicle while waiting for core cooling and application of the aortic
cross-clamp. The anesthesiologist has just started playing the overture to "Swan
Lake" and you are settling down for what should be a pleasant few hours, when
your perfusionist intrudes upon this idyll saying that he cannot maintain a perfusion
pressure over 30 mmHg and during these few horrifying seconds his cardiotomy
reservoir is overflowing.

M. E. Lee
Department of Cardiac Surgery, Centinela Hospital Medical Center, Inglewood, CA, USA

T. M. Sundt (✉)
Division of Cardiac Surgery, Massachusetts General Hospital, Boston, MA, USA
e-mail: tsundt@mgh.harvard.edu

© The Author(s), under exclusive license to Springer Nature Switzerland AG 2022
T. M. Sundt et al. (eds.), *Near Misses in Cardiac Surgery*,
https://doi.org/10.1007/978-3-030-92750-9_49

Solution

Since the heart is empty, you know there cannot be a problem with impaired venous return. The ascending aorta appears normal, and the anesthesiologist confirms there is no aortic dissection apparent on ECHO. As you turn around to look at the amazing site in the oxygenator, the perfusionist spots the problem: You have neglected to clamp the recirculation shunt between the arterial and venous lines, a step performed back at the pump in your home hospital. You quickly grab the tubing clamp, apply it to the line, grateful to see the perfusion pressure rise as the level in the oxygenator falls, and the curtain rises on Act 1 of "Swan Lake." At this point you feel like an unwelcome guest at Siegfried's birthday party, although the remainder of your case proceeds as you had originally intended.

Discussion

The frequency with which cardiopulmonary bypass is conducted in the current era can lead to a false sense of simplicity. In fact, the conduct of cardiopulmonary bypass is a complex undertaking requiring coordination amongst multiple individuals of diverse educational backgrounds dealing with a remarkably sophisticated machine which has been improved to the point of near 6 Sigma performance. It is indeed ideally "routine" which is to say a sequence of actions that is regularly followed according to a standard program. As such it is critical that those steps be conducted correctly and that communication amongst caregivers be effective.

If one accepts the premise that human error is responsible for most complications relating to cardiopulmonary bypass rather than equipment malfunction, then it becomes apparent that consistently excellent results demand attention to principles of cognitive psychology and human factors science. Fundamental to the conduct of a complex procedure, such as the conduct of cardiopulmonary bypass, is the need to recognize the limitations of the individual human mind, including the potential for task overload and the necessity for all members of the team to have the same shared mental model and situational awareness. Given the limitations of carbon-based life forms, standardization of protocols and processes is an obvious approach to reducing cognitive workload and makes it easier for everyone to be on the same page. Similarly, equipment setup should be standardized at a minimum within a given institution and ideally within an entire practice. In this case you were thrown off because of a seemingly trivial difference in preference for perfusion practice. There is nothing trivial about extracorporeal circulation.

A standardized protocol in process ensures that all members of the heart team will function in concert, using similar approaches to monitoring, techniques of anesthesia, instrument trays, and perfusion. It also means the patterns of interaction amongst the anesthesiologist, surgeon, perfusionist, and nurse remain constant and predictable from case to case. Communication is critical to teamwork and teamwork is critical to success. The practice of "read back—speak back" ensures that what was said was heard and that what was heard is what was said. The administration of anesthetic agents and vasoactive drugs during bypass must be called out between the anesthesiologist and the perfusionist. The anesthesiologist must know to lower the blood pressure before the aortic cannulation and be prepared to elevate it in anticipation of retrograde autologous prime. The perfusionist must lower the perfusion pressure in anticipation of aortic cross clamping and unclamping. The scrub nurse should know enough about every procedure to anticipate the next step and thereby maintain the fluid rhythm created by the swift, silent passage of instruments from one hand to the other. Disruptions in the flow of the operation have been demonstrated to lead to technical failures.

While there are downsides to checklists, this is an ideal time for their implementation. This is in fact a perfect example of an ideal circumstance for the implementation of checklists—where a sequence of events needs to occur in precisely the same order and same way every time, like the notes of a symphony, in order to reach a pre-ordained conclusion. Both initiation of cardiopulmonary bypass and weaning from bypass are examples. Checklists are particularly effective when dealing with a human machine interface, which is essentially what this process entails. Industrial engineers identify "single-point vulnerabilities" where critical irreversible errors may occur. Commencement of cardiopulmonary bypass without administering heparin, or weaning from bypass without activating the anesthesia ventilator, are two examples of such errors that can and have led to unnecessary fatalities. Both can be prevented with adherence to a brief but thoughtful checklist. Other applications of checklists include the anesthesiologist in the preoperative check of his machine and preparation of drugs and the perfusionist in setting up the pump oxygenator.

Preoperative briefings are also important at times when specific details of the particular patient in the particular case can be reviewed with the team to anticipate the overall arc of the case. In contrast to checklists, which are the same every time, briefings should be unique and different every time, tailored to the specific patient and the specific procedure.

The importance of each discipline having a basic awareness of what should be happening at a given time and being willing to communicate any irregularity in the sequence of events constitutes a system of checks and balances that is the essence of teamwork and is the key to minimal morbidity and mortality.

Bibliography

1. Wahr JA, Prager RL, Abernathy JH 3rd, Martinez EA, Salas E, Seifert PC, Groom RC, Spiess BD, Searles BE, Sundt TM 3rd, Sanchez JA, Shappell SA, Culig MH, Lazzara EH, Fitzgerald DC, Thourani VH, Eghtesady P, Ikonomidis JS, England MR, Sellke FW, Nussmeier NA. Patient safety in the cardiac operating room: human factors and teamwork: a scientific statement from the American Heart Association American Heart Association Council on Cardiovascular Surgery and Anesthesia, council on cardiovascular and stroke nursing, and council on quality of care and outcomes research. Circulation. 2013;128(10):1139–69. https://doi.org/10.1161/CIR.0b013e3182a38efa Epub 2013 Aug 5 PMID: 2391825.
2. Wiegmann DA, ElBardissi AW, Dearani JA, Daly RC, Sundt TM 3rd. Disruptions in surgical flow and their relationship to surgical errors: an exploratory investigation. Surgery. 2007;142 (5):658–65. https://doi.org/10.1016/j.surg.2007.07.034 PMID: 17981185.
3. Henrickson SE, Wadhera RK, Elbardissi AW, Wiegmann DA, Sundt TM 3rd. Development and pilot evaluation of a preoperative briefing protocol for cardiovascular surgery. J Am Coll Surg. 2009;208(6):1115–23. https://doi.org/10.1016/j.jamcollsurg.2009.01.037 Epub 2009 Apr 17 PMID: 19476900.

Chapter 50
Debriding "Candle Wax Calcification"

Jordan P. Bloom and David A. D'Alessandro

Problem

You are thrilled to be doing an isolated surgical aortic valve replacement as an early start second case. It has been a long week and you are eager to get out in time to pick up flowers for your spouse recognizing that they have been late nights for them too. The patient is a 58-year-old man with bicuspid aortic stenosis. You cannulate the ascending aorta, place a dual stage cannula in the right atrium, and place an antegrade cardioplegia cannula. Without aortic regurgitation you are comfortable forgoing a retrograde cannula. After diastolic cardioplegic arrest, you open the aorta and find a severely calcified aortic valve with fusion of the right and left coronary leaflets. Much to your chagrin, the aorta is not dilated at all. In fact, the sinotubular junction is calcified as well, making exposure challenging. As you carefully debride the annulus in the non-coronary sinus with the pituitary rongeur, you encounter a heavy bar of calcium extending down the anterior leaflet of the mitral valve. While you could potentially place your valve sutures above this bar, it is unpleasant looking and you think might restrict the mobility of the mitral valve leaflet, so you carefully remove it using the rongeur. The valve prosthesis seats nicely and the remainder of the procedure is uneventful. The patient easily separates from cardiopulmonary bypass on no inotropes and you are anticipating a lovely evening when, just as you are getting ready to decannulate the patient, your eagle-eyed anesthesiologist notifies you that there is a high velocity jet of mitral regurgitation by transesophageal echocardiography. In disbelief you ask the echocardiographer if they have the gain adjusted correctly.

J. P. Bloom · D. A. D'Alessandro (✉)
Department of Surgery, Massachusetts General Hospital, Boston, MA, USA
e-mail: dadalessandro@mgh.harvard.edu

J. P. Bloom
e-mail: jpbloom@mgh.harvard.edu

© The Author(s), under exclusive license to Springer Nature Switzerland AG 2022   199
T. M. Sundt et al. (eds.), *Near Misses in Cardiac Surgery*,
https://doi.org/10.1007/978-3-030-92750-9_50

Solution

After careful review, the location of the jet is on the anterior leaflet of the mitral valve, just under the left coronary cusp. You recognize that it must be related to your efforts to decalcify the anterior leaflet. You consider the options for repair. Fortunately, the patient chose a tissue prosthesis making repair through the prosthesis an option. Concerned that you might damage the valve though, neutralizing almost all that you have done up to now, you re-arrest the heart and explore the mitral valve via a standard left atriotomy. Unfortunately, the exposure is quite limited by the incompressible aortic prothesis and you cannot see the base of the anterior leaflet. The option of converting to a transeptal atrial incision crosses your mind but would require weaning from bypass and converting to bicaval cannulation. With some degree of apprehension, you reopen the aortotomy and work through the prosthesis. Using a fine right angle clamp you identify the perforation and proceed to repair it primarily. Glancing up at the clock in the OR you are a bit disappointed to see that florist is closed, but you are grateful that so it the hole in the valve.

Discussion

When debriding calcium for an aortic valve replacement, one must take caution in over debriding the annulus. The objective is to prepare the annulus to accommodate the prosthesis and to facilitate annular suture placement. The mantra which has been applied to mitral annular calcification "respectfully resect" also applies to the aortic annulus in this scenario. Very commonly there is calcium which extends downward from the annulus in the region of the commissure between the left and non-coronary sinuses and the non-coronary sinuses of Valsalva down the anterior leaflet of the mitral valve just as candlewax runs down a candlestick. There is diversity of opinion regarding the necessity to debride with some arguing that it may impair anterior leaflet motion while others argue as minimalist approach to remove only what is necessary to seat the valve. If the calcium is excessive or the surgeon feels they must debride this calcium, it should be done with the utmost caution to avoid injury to the mitral valve. If there is concern for injury, the leaflet can be gently probed with a blunt nerve hook. If the hole in the mitral valve is small, it may be able to be repaired primarily, however a small autologous pericardial patch is strongly recommended when possible in the interest of reducing tension and enhancing durability.

Bibliography

1. Sareyyupoglu B, et al. Safety and durability of mitral valve repair for anterior leaflet perforation. The J Thorac Cardiovasc Surg. 2010;139:1488–93.
2. Maddali MM, Waje ND, Kandachar PS, Ajmi WAAAA, Mohamed B. Rare cause of new mitral regurgitation after aortic valve replacement. J Cardiothorac Vasc Anesth. 2016;30:845–7.
3. Kadirogullari E, Onan B, Guler S, Erkanli K. Perforation of the anterior mitral leaflet after aortic valve replacement with root enlargement. The Ann Thorac Surg. 2017;104:e345–6.
4. Pezzella AT, Utley JR, VanderSalm TJ. Operative approaches to the left atrium and mitral valve: an update. Oper Tech Thorac Cardiac Surg. 1998;3:74–94.

Index

© The Editor(s) (if applicable) and The Author(s), under exclusive license to
Springer Nature Switzerland AG 2022
T. M. Sundt et al. (eds.), *Near Misses in Cardiac Surgery*,
https://doi.org/10.1007/978-3-030-92750-9

Printed in the United States
by Baker & Taylor Publisher Services